Editor:
Dr Liam Brennan

AVINASH ASWATH

Guide to the FRCA examination
The Final

Third Edition
September 2011

ISBN 1-900936-31-3

Design and layout by The Royal College of Anaesthetists.

Contents

Introduction 5

Section 1: Examination Structure and Guidance

Short answer questions	9
Multiple choice questions	13
Final FRCA Structured Oral Examination (SOE)	16
Clinical anaesthesia SOE	17
Clinical science SOE	23
Examination guidance	28
Appendix A: FRCA Examination changes	30

Section 2: Questions

SAQ examination	
SAQ Paper 1	35
SAQ Paper 2	38
MCQ examination	
Multiple True or False (MTF)	41
Single Best Answer (SBA)	87
SOE examination	
Clinical Anaesthesia – Long Cases	101
Clinical Anaesthesia – Short Cases	110
Clinical Science	114

Section 3: Answers

SAQ examination	
SAQ Paper 1	119
SAQ Paper 2	136
MCQ examination	
Multiple True or False (MTF)	155
Single Best Answer (SBA)	193
SOE examination	
Clinical Anaesthesia – Long Cases	211
Clinical Anaesthesia – Short Cases	217
Clinical Science	227

Introduction

Dr Liam Brennan, Member of Council and Chairman,
Final FRCA Examination

Since the last edition of this guide was published in 2008, the Final FRCA examination has undergone some significant changes (summarised in Appendix A). The new CCT curriculum introduced in 2010 has been a major impetus. All examination questions will be blueprinted against the new curriculum from September 2011. It is therefore timely to produce a new edition of the Final exam guide which includes examples of the most contemporary examination material, including single best answer MCQ questions (SBAs). We hope that it will help candidates (and their trainers) appreciate the breadth and depth of the examination and the expected standard of answers.

Examiners are commonly asked why does the content and structure of the exam need to change. The FRCA examinations are but one of a range of tools used to assess progress of trainees through the CCT curriculum. The GMC, as our regulator, requires the College to produce a fair, reliable and suitably robust examination that reflects best contemporary assessment practice. Consequently we have established a modular structure with uncoupling of the written from the oral components of the examination, instituted a numeric marking system and introduced SBAs as an alternative genre of MCQ question. No doubt the examination will undergo further changes in the future. However, candidates and trainers are assured that the College guarantees that modifications will only be introduced following careful consideration and with adequate notice.

As in previous editions, the guide is in three parts. In Section 1 current Chairmen of each of the relevant Sub Groups describe their component of the Final examination including details of the marking system and standard setting. There is also a summary of the revised process for candidates who request guidance from the College due to difficulties in passing the examinations. In Section 2 are examples of questions taken from the current bank of questions and, finally, in Section 3 are the answers and some explanation.

I would like to take this opportunity, on behalf of the Council of The Royal College of Anaesthetists, to thank all those examiners and members of the College Exams Department who have contributed so much to the Examination and to this guide. Their tireless efforts have ensured that the FRCA examinations maintain the highest standards for the benefit of patients and are a key factor in ensuring the respect in which our specialty is held by the whole medical community.

DIVINUM SEDARE DOLOREM

Section 1: Examination Structure and Guidance

Short answer questions

Dr David Noble, Chairman, SAQ Sub Group

The aim of the SAQ paper is to test higher thinking including: judgement, the ability to prioritise and summarise, and the capability to present an argument clearly and succinctly in writing. It complements the MCQ and oral examinations which test other knowledge-based competences of presenting candidates. The examiners recognise that written assessments are arduous, but the College believes it is still appropriate to continue to use this form of examining technique. It is reassuring to note that the statistical techniques which are used to evaluate the SAQ paper demonstrate that this section of the Final FRCA is consistently an appropriately reliable test which compares favourably with the other examination methods used, notably the MCQ and SOEs.

The format of the SAQ paper has changed little since the last edition of the exam guide was published, with two important exceptions. Previously, two marks (10% of the total mark for each question) were awarded for 'judgement, prioritisation and clarity' of the answer. From the March 2011 diet of the examination this discretionary element of the SAQ mark will no longer feature in the marking schedule and credit will be awarded solely on the basis of the content of the answer. From the same diet of the exam, the regulation allowing for deduction of up to two marks for 'unsafe' answers will also be abandoned. The Final examining board have made these changes to decrease the subjectivity in SAQ marking and so improve the overall reliability of the examination.

Setting the paper

Constructing the SAQ paper is time-consuming and requires much thought and discussion. A diverse range of questions sampling the whole of the curriculum should be included. The questions must allow time for analytical thought, and the paper must determine and maintain the College's standards.

In addition to specific knowledge-based competences listed within the intermediate curriculum additional sources of examination material may be developed from guidance or recommendations published by healthcare organisations such as RCoA, AAGBI, NCEPOD, NICE, NPSA, CEMACH, etc. The public expects their doctors to keep up to date with important developments and such material may be examined under the collective umbrella of 'professionalism', which is detailed in Annex A of the CCT in Anaesthetics curriculum 2010. Candidates should also remember that knowledge gained during the basic units of training, including the clinical sciences, may also be required to answer SAQ questions satisfactorily.

Examiners are asked to submit questions several months in advance and the SAQ Sub Group select the final 12 bearing in mind the aim of each question and the balance of the paper as a whole. Each question is reviewed and refined several times with the intention of making the purpose of the question as clear as possible.

Marking guides are provided for the examiners and these are also checked and rechecked against the question. No question is accepted where the marking guide runs to more than one page. Within this third edition of the guide the answers for paper 1 are the templates actually used by the examiners for the March 2011 examination. Questions in paper 2 are taken from older papers and the answer template has been modified to reflect the new marking schema (i.e. with no discretionary marks).

Answering SAQ questions

Candidates are advised to read the paper carefully. Every word in each question is there for a purpose, and the questions should be answered by providing no more and no less than what is asked. Where, for example, a question asks about pre-operative management, no marks will be given for operative or post-operative management. If a question says 'list' then a list is what is required.

Examiners are keen that candidates' answers should be concise and suitably focused. Candidates who find that they are writing much more than two pages are likely to be missing the point. The answer should not be so narrow to omit relevant, scoring material or contain large amounts of irrelevant information. Skill at prioritising the elements to include in SAQ answers only develops with practice, ideally under simulated exam conditions.

It is recommended that candidates should consider the content of their answer for several minutes and then write for 10–12 minutes. The examiners have given careful thought as to how much is expected in response to each question to ensure it is achievable in the time allocated. Timing is crucial and candidates will not be maximising their chances of passing if they spend too much time on some questions and leave too little time to score adequately on others.

Whenever possible, questions are broken down into sub-sections. Percentage marks allocated to each section are indicated and candidates are strongly advised to allocate their time appropriately. For example if a sub-section commands 10% of the marks available, a superbly comprehensive answer to that part can only realise two marks and no more.

Two questions should be answered in each of the six answer books provided to each candidate. One question is printed on the first page and the second halfway through the answer book. Candidates should start each question on the relevant page and indicate clearly the sub-section of the question they are answering. It is essential that candidates use the correct answer book for each question. Failure to do so may result in a candidate being deemed to have not completed the SAQ paper correctly and therefore to fail the written examination.

Finally, although marks are not deducted for poor handwriting, candidates should realise that examiners cannot award marks for material they cannot read so please ensure that you write legibly.

Standard setting

Approximately six weeks before the written examination, the examiners meet in teams and go over the two questions they are to mark. They refine the marking schedule further and discuss a preliminary pass mark for each question. Currently, about six to eight examiners will share the marking of each pair of questions. Six examiners will therefore participate in marking any individual candidate's SAQ paper. Increasing the number of markers involved in assessing each candidate's paper reduces the effect of any variability between examiners. Soon after the written examination, at a standard setting meeting, the examiners mark several specimen answers in their groups to calibrate their marking and verify the final version of the marking guide. Hence every effort is made to make the marking as uniform between examiners as possible.

Marking

Each SAQ is now marked out of 20 using the marking guide finally decided by the examiners. The pass mark for each question is agreed by the examiners before they mark the papers; this is based on their expectation of what a borderline candidate who is just at the pass standard should achieve. (This process is known as modified Angoff referencing.) Questions span varying degrees of difficulty and so pass marks for different questions vary accordingly. Typically pass marks range from 11 to 14 out of 20 marks. The 'examiner generated' pass marks for the 12 questions are summed to give a total pass mark for the whole paper.

To allow for variation in the examination's reliability this mark is then reduced by one standard error of the mean to give the actual pass mark that is used for the SAQ paper. This mark is then combined with the pass mark for the MCQ paper to give the overall pass mark for the written examination.

Each examiner will have approximately 60-80 books to mark (120–160 answers). At the time of marking the examiners will note information that is correct, incorrect, apparently confusing or questionable and will note omissions against the marking guide. They will allocate marks to each section of the question and, having completed marking the whole question, will add up the total.

Quality assurance

Once marking is completed all of the marks are checked for arithmetic errors and any ambiguities in the marking. The performance of each question and the paper as a whole are scrutinised in detail and subjected to statistical analyses to determine reliability. Questions that have low pass rates are looked at more closely to ascertain if there are any reasons to account for the poor performance. Examiners provide their comments on each question and identify any common themes in candidates' performance. The Chair of the SAQ group produces a report on the performance of each SAQ paper which is published on the RCoA website for the benefit of candidates and trainers.

Summary

Candidates who have prepared thoroughly and have adequate experience of anaesthesia, intensive care medicine and pain management, together with a solid knowledge of basic sciences, will have the best chance in the SAQ examination.

Currently, most questions used for the SAQ examination are newly created for that particular sitting. However questions may be repeated and one or more may be used in any SAQ paper. This may become an increasing feature as a question bank is built up. There are many reasons for this but two important aspects are to facilitate a more balanced paper and to drive learning. Candidates are expected to be familiar with recent important reports and guidelines. They are advised to practise an SAQ paper under examination conditions as, for many, it will be several years since they have written a three-hour paper.

Finally, the most important advice is repeated. Read the question carefully, answer it no more and no less and pay strict attention to timing.

Multiple choice questions

Dr Tim Smith, Chairman, Final FRCA MCQ Sub Group
Dr Liam Brennan, Chairman, Final FRCA Examination

The Final Examination MCQ paper comprises 90 stems to be completed in three hours. It is divided into two sections with 60 multiple-true-false (MTF) and 30 single-best answer (SBA) questions.

Since the introduction of SBAs to the exam in September 2010, the construct of the MCQ paper is as follows:

Twenty MTF questions in medicine and surgery, 20 MTF questions in applied basic science (including clinical measurement), 15 MTF questions in intensive care medicine, 5 MTF questions in pain management.

Twenty SBA questions in clinical anaesthesia, 5 SBA questions in intensive care medicine, 5 SBA questions in pain management.

The Examiners from the MCQ Sub Group are responsible for a databank of over a thousand questions covering all aspects of the curriculum – identified by an 'E' (Examination) in the document 'The CCT in Anaesthetics Training Programme', August 2010. Although most of the questions relate to subject areas covered in the intermediate curriculum, candidates are reminded that the Final exam may include questions related to the basic level curriculum (including basic sciences) and professionalism in medical practice (Annex A of the CCT document). New questions are constantly being developed and existing questions modified by the examiners so as to make the question bank reflect the breadth of the curriculum.

The MTF section is primarily a test of factual knowledge. Each MTF question stem has five items; each item can be true or false. All the questions are equally valuable with a correct answer scoring +1, and an incorrect answer or unanswered question scoring zero. It is possible for all five parts of a question to be 'true' or indeed for all five parts to be 'false'.

However, the MTF style of question does not allow facts to be placed in context, or lend itself to testing the application of knowledge and problem solving that is so essential in clinical practice. This is where SBAs are invaluable; they allow the candidate to demonstrate that they 'know how' rather than simply 'know' thus assessing a higher level of understanding.

SBAs consist of a stem, lead-in question and five options. The stem is a clinical vignette in clinical anaesthesia, intensive care or pain medicine (acute or chronic). The stem has a maximum of 60 words focusing on a single problem. The lead-in is short and precise and poses a single question. The five options are all possible solutions or responses to the question arising from the stem. However, one of the options will be the best response, and the remaining four will be inferior. A useful approach for candidates is to read the stem and lead-in question while covering up the five options so that they cannot be seen. The answer that occurs to a well-prepared candidate at this stage, and then appears in the list of options, is likely to be the correct best response. Candidates make a single mark on their answer sheet next to their choice for each question. Four marks are scored for each correct answer. This mark is based on the premise that a candidate needs to discount four options in order to arrive at the single, best answer. If candidates make more than one response to a question then no marks will be awarded for that question.

As there is no negative marking in the MCQ exam, it is in your interests to answer every question and every option. To leave out answers means that you lose out on the possibility of getting the answer right and the mark that goes with it!

The pass mark varies slightly with each diet of the exam in order to reflect the inevitable variation in difficulty of a particular exam. The overall pass mark for the MCQ since the introduction of SBAs is around 70–75%. The MCQ Core Group meets approximately one week after the MCQ examination to set the pass mark. Prior to this meeting, 'Angoff referencing' is performed. In this process around 20 examiners are given the paper (without the answers) and each independently decides for every question the probability of the borderline candidate knowing the correct answer. This process of criterion referencing has been shown to have a high validity in determining the pass standard and helps to ensure that your examination is both fair and reliable.

It is recommended that you mark your answers on the question paper and transfer them to the optical mark reader (OMR) sheets, using the pencil provided, when you have completed the paper and you are sure about your answers. You can change your answer on the OMR sheet, ensuring that you erase the incorrect response and indicate the new answer with a firm pencil mark. However you choose to mark your OMR sheet please make sure that you allow sufficient time to transcribe your answers and mark them firmly. Transcription errors are all too easy to make if rushed. Please be aware that extra time will not be allowed for transcribing answers to the OMR sheet.

You will need a broad knowledge of the curriculum to pass the MCQ examination. Answering the practice questions will help you become familiar with the style of the exam and the level of knowledge required. The questions included in this guide may have been asked previously or are adapted from those that are currently in the question bank. However, candidates are reminded that questions are constantly under review and small modifications may change the character of the question and thus the answers. There is, therefore, little to be gained from simply memorising the answers to the questions published in this guide. You should therefore regard these practice questions as a valuable part of your exam preparation but will, of itself, not be sufficient to guarantee an overall pass.

Final FRCA Structured Oral Examination (SOE)

The Structured Oral Examination (SOE) is a stand-alone component of the Final FRCA Examination. Success in the Final FRCA written examination (in the preceding two years) is required before you may enter the SOE. A maximum of six attempts at the SOE are permitted.

The SOE is comprised of two sections:

1 Clinical Anaesthesia

2 Clinical Science

Clinical anaesthesia SOE

Dr Platon Razis, Chairman, Clinical Anaesthesia Sub Group
Dr Michael Tremlett, Short Case Lead, Clinical Anaesthesia Sub Group

Aim of the SOE in Clinical Anaesthesia

The Final FRCA examination is an assessment of the knowledge trainees are expected to have acquired in completing the Intermediate Level of training towards a CCT in Anaesthetics. The sub-section in Clinical Anaesthesia complements workplace-based assessments to examine in a standardised format the understanding and theoretical application of this knowledge in clinical practice. It requires the candidate to appreciate the anaesthetic significance of clinical situations and demonstrate correct interpretation of clinical investigations in the planning of optimal peri-operative anaesthetic care. As this is often a question of judgement, as long as the candidate supports their chosen management options with well reasoned discussion based on sound scientific principles, the examiners will be satisfied. For that reason, all examiners in the Final FRCA have at least three years' experience as an examiner in the Primary FRCA before moving to the Final Examination. In preparing the questions every effort is made to sample widely from the curriculum and minimise repetition of topics between the two sections of the SOE examination.

Structure of the SOE in Clinical Anaesthesia

The Clinical Anaesthesia examination is 50 minutes long and is the first section of the SOE each candidate will face. Candidates are ushered into a room where they are given ten minutes to review the outline of a clinical long case and any associated investigations. Candidates should use the review time wisely and make notes that they can take to the examination table. Although the long cases vary, candidates are likely to be asked about the pre-operative issues (including co-morbidities) that will influence peri-operative management, plans for how you will conduct the anaesthetic and a third section which may include discussion of post-operative care. Candidates should also be aware that some of the long cases may relate to intensive care practice and pain medicine. At the end of the review period, candidates are escorted into the examination room where they have been assigned to an examination table with a pair of examiners. One of the examiners will question the candidate for 20 minutes focusing on the long case and then hand over to their co-examiner who will examine the candidate for 20 minutes on three unrelated short cases. There may also be a third person at the table observing the examination process. This may be a College Tutor, Regional Advisor or another examiner who is 'auditing' the examiners, but will not in any way take part in the assessment process. Occasionally, a candidate will know one of the examiners or the visitor at their table. If this occurs, the candidate should indicate the problem immediately before the examination commences and the invigilator will immediately assign the candidate to another table.

Bells mark the beginning and end of all SOEs and the examiners and College staff will direct the candidates appropriately. The clinical SOEs are undertaken in the morning which is divided into four time slots, with all candidates in each cohort being examined on the same material. The examiners' questions are guided by an outline which includes standard opening questions. The intention is that all candidates should have a similar SOE, irrespective of the examiners they face.

The long case

The long case is based on a real patient with copies of the original investigations from the case. It will consist of an outline history including relevant drug therapy, key clinical examination findings and investigations. Usually there will be a chest radiograph, though sometimes there is a different radiological investigation such as a CT or MRI scan. Although this is not a radiology examination, candidates will need to give an opinion on the radiographs at a level expected of them in their clinical practice. The same applies to blood tests, ECGs lung function tests, echocardiograms etc. In preparing for the SOE candidates should develop a technique for examining investigations methodically, although because of time constraints they will often be asked to point out the salient features. The presence of an investigation does not mean that it is abnormal as it is equally important in clinical practice to recognise when tests are normal. Candidates are expected to construct an overview of the clinical problems taking into account important findings, decide what further information and investigations they would like to obtain, and consider the management options. They do not need to commit the results to memory as there are copies of all the material at the examination table for reference. Candidates are encouraged to make notes during the ten minute review of the material which can be taken through to the examination table. The cases are often complex to allow the examiner enough scope to examine the excellent candidates without running out of material, or to move on to other areas should weaker candidates become stuck. The level of questioning will reflect the expected experience of the average candidate who is a year 3 or 4 specialty registrar.

Once candidates are settled at the exam table, a bell will sound and one of the examiners will start examining on the long case; the other examiner will listen and make notes of their responses. The examiner will usually begin by asking for a brief overview of the case, which should be kept concise, as a more in-depth discussion will follow. For example:

This is a case of a 60-year-old man scheduled for an elective laparoscopic cholecystectomy who has a history of severe chronic obstructive airway disease as demonstrated by the lung function tests and arterial blood gases. Surgery should be delayed as he has a chest infection, and an HDU bed should be available for post-operative care when he is well enough to proceed.

This is a broad overview that leaves a lot of detail for further discussion which the examiner can explore over the ensuing 20 minutes. The long case should be like a discussion between professionals as to the best way to proceed. When asked how to manage a particular situation, candidates should not be afraid to voice an opinion but must be prepared to justify their choice. There is quite often no right or wrong answer but a number of alternatives each of which have their pros and cons. The examiners want to see the candidates using their judgement to arrive at a decision, and are not necessarily looking for a particular answer. For example, candidates often mention fibreoptic intubation for any problem involving an airway concern, but this may be inappropriate in the presence of bleeding or unhelpful for a subglottic problem. It is accepted that candidates will not have experience of some of these situations, but a sensible application of safe basic principles will be sufficient to satisfy the examiners.

The long case is divided into three sections, although the examiner may move on to each section without the candidate being aware of it. If this is an operative case it may break down into pre-, intra- and post-operative care but may not. There is often a critical incident included as part of the discussion, with further investigations if appropriate. As each section is marked separately and independently by each examiner, it is important to remain positive in answering each question, as a poor performance in one section could be offset by good answers in the other two.

The short clinical cases

There are three Short Clinical Cases which may cover any aspect of practice as defined in the Intermediate Curriculum. Each short case will last about seven minutes and the examiner will move from one topic to the next ensuring that adequate time is allocated to display the necessary knowledge and understanding in each area. The combination of one long case and three short cases allows us to examine across the breadth of the curriculum. Candidates should therefore expect to be questioned on a range of topics covering not only General Units of Training but also aspects of the knowledge base of Additional and Key units of Training (the practice of intensive care medicine, pain management and cardiac, neuro-, paediatric and obstetric anaesthesia).

The short cases will be framed from a clinical perspective which will aim to realistically reflect clinical practice. For instance it is unlikely candidates will be asked directly to list the problems of anaesthesia for the patient in atrial fibrillation as this is a test of pure knowledge best covered in the written papers. Instead a scenario will be described where a patient has been seen in pre-assessment and an ECG has been undertaken. This will be shown to the candidate who will have to identify atrial fibrillation and will then explore its relevance in a specific clinical situation and the options for management. It is therefore important in preparing for the clinical SOEs that candidates develop a systematic approach to interpretation of investigations and are able to easily recognise common abnormalities.

Similarly we will not ask as an opening question about how to manage a patient with, for example aortic stenosis. Instead, we will present a case in which a patient with a femoral neck fracture on the trauma list is found to have a systolic murmur, and explore how you would proceed with the clinical management.

That said, there are occasions when we may define the clinical condition and ask its anaesthetic relevance. Almost always in clinical practice you would know a patient has Down's Syndrome before you meet them, and it is then appropriate to ask the clinical implications of this underlying diagnosis in a child presenting say for adenotonsillectomy. Again this mirrors real clinical practice.

Everyone being examined at the same time will be asked about the same Clinical Cases. The examiners have a sheet describing the areas they are to explore with each Clinical Short Case. In practice after the opening question, the SOE may progress slightly differently on different tables. The supplementary questions each examiner asks after the common opening question will in part be determined by the answer to the initial question. It is by this semi-structured series of predominately open questions that we can explore whether candidates truly have understanding as well as knowledge.

Examples of typical short clinical questions with the likely answers are included later in this booklet.

Marking

As each examiner marks independently, they will each award three separate scores for the three sections of the long case and one score for each of the three short cases. The candidate will therefore have six separate scores from each examiner making a total of 12 scores. Each individual score will be 0, 1 or 2 based on the following assessment:

0 = The candidate showed very limited knowledge or understanding of the topic

1 = The candidate showed incomplete/partial knowledge or understanding of the topic

2 = The candidate showed satisfactory knowledge and understanding of the topic

There is therefore a possible maximum of 24 marks for the SOE in Clinical Anaesthesia. An example of a possible mark sheet of the two examiners combined is given below.

Candidate 666	**Examiner A**	**Examiner B**
Long Case:		
Pre-operative assessment	2	2
Intra-operative care	2	2
Post-operative care/Critical Incident	2	2
Short Cases:		
Case 1	2	2
Case 2	0	0
Case 3	2	2
Total = 20/24	**10**	**10**

The pass mark for the overall SOE examination is 32 marks. Therefore despite the poor scores in one of the short cases the candidate can still afford to drop up to four further marks in the Clinical Science SOE and still pass. This means that as no single section or short case is sufficient to fail the examination outright, the candidate must treat each section separately and start afresh even if they have answered the preceding question poorly.

Preparing for the SOE in Clinical Anaesthesia

As this part of the examination aims to replicate clinical practice, preparation should consist of the assessment and planning for anaesthesia of the patients you manage every day. For example, if you see a diabetic patient presenting as an urgent case with a hip fracture then read up the peri-operative care of patients with diabetes. Learn from the surgeon the choices of surgical treatment available, the reasons a specific course has been chosen and the associated surgical risks and complications. Present the case to a consultant colleague if you are being supervised. Systematically go through the investigations and describe what they show and explain how this may influence your management. List the choices of anaesthetic management available and the advantages and disadvantages of each, and then describe what you would actually do.

Match your learning to the current training module as learning neuro-anaesthesia, for example, is much easier to understand and remember when you are actually doing it. In addition, you should map learning to the curriculum, as although you cannot expect to see everything, basic knowledge and understanding of important but less common problems is required. It is therefore advisable not to take the examination too soon, and to ensure that you have a broad experience of the major sub-specialities before applying to sit the SOE.

In the SOE examination, be clear and succinct. The ability to quickly evaluate clinical problems and communicate your conclusions effectively is an important component of adequate performance. In deciding on a course of action, base your answer on what you would really do and do not be tempted to try and second guess the examiner. Although safety is paramount, a common sense approach which weighs up the alternatives is important. If your answer to every airway problem is an awake fibreoptic intubation, we may doubt your credibility as a practising anaesthetist!

We do not expect you to have seen and done everything. However, we do expect that you have the knowledge, judgement and first-hand experience of the majority of the Intermediate Curriculum. In deciding whether a candidate has achieved the required standard, we commonly apply the 'Trainee Test' i.e. if we were on-call together and were discussing a case on the telephone, would we be convinced that not only did you appreciate the problems surrounding the case, but that you had a sensible anaesthetic plan which you could communicate effectively to theatre staff and surgeons. As an anaesthetist we often find ourselves acting as the patient's advocate. Our role as examiners is to ensure that on behalf of the general public, candidates have demonstrated adequate knowledge and understanding of the professional requirements needed to fulfil that role.

Clinical science SOE

Dr Adrian Pearce, Chairman, Clinical Science Sub Group

The Clinical Science oral is intended to test a candidate's understanding of basic medical science as applied to the practice of clinical anaesthesia, intensive care and acute and chronic pain management. In the morning long and short cases you are presented with clinical scenarios and will be examined on the clinical care of the patient. In the afternoon you are tested on the knowledge that underpins those professional judgements and your clinical practice. This knowledge is mostly basic science but may include published guidelines and other topics within healthcare management. The areas covered in the clinical science examination are shown in the CCT document. You have already been examined on your fundamental understanding of basic medical science in the Primary Examination and there is no reason to repeat this. The Final Fellowship examination is much more concerned with testing how this knowledge base informs and supports your clinical decision-making in everyday practice.

There has been substantial change in the clinical science questions over the last few years. They now all start with a clinically orientated opening question before a more detailed testing of underlying knowledge. It may not always be clear always from the opening question which of the four core science disciplines (clinical measurement, physiology, pharmacology and anatomy) is being examined. For example an opening question asking the candidate to list the intra-operative anaesthetic problems during scoliosis surgery may lead on to monitoring of spinal cord function (Clinical measurement), the blood supply of the spinal cord (Anatomy) , effects of the prone position (Physiology) or even more detailed knowledge of drugs used in a wake-up test (Pharmacology). Whilst the answer to the opening question is independent of the nature of the supplementary questions, we believe that it will be fairest if you are alerted early to which discipline is involved and the examiner may start by announcing this.

A development already introduced in the clinical anaesthesia SOEs is the use of a computer screen at the examining table to display relevant radiology or other artefacts. With prior notification to candidates, the same technology may also be used to enrich the clinical science orals in the future. For example, anatomy diagrams, ultrasound pictures, photographs of equipment or data capture might be displayed on the computer screens to complement the examiner's question.

Your oral will be conducted by examiners who are all practising clinicians with a vast experience of all aspects of anaesthesia, intensive care and pain management. Many have been examining in Fellowship examinations for a considerable time and all are involved in postgraduate teaching.

The oral

Each examiner is provided with the topics to be discussed and guidance notes as illustrated later in this book. It is important to understand that, although the same topic is being examined simultaneously for each cohort of candidates that enter the exam room, no two orals will be identical. The intention is to establish a dialogue between the candidate and the examiner with the candidate doing most of the talking. The opening and supplementary questions are scripted to make the examination equitable but the guidance notes are only illustrative. The direction of the oral can depend upon the responses given by the candidate, especially if the examiner wishes to explore further something the candidate has said. There are no traps, catches or hidden agendas in any of the questions.

On arrival in the examination room you will be directed to the correct table by a member of the examinations staff. If you know one of the examiners because they are currently or have been involved with your training in the past please do not sit down and you will be re-directed to a new table. At your table the examiners will check your candidate number. The Clinical Science oral is 30 minutes long comprising two 15-minute sessions; you will be examined by two examiners in turn. A bell will ring to indicate the start of the oral and after 15 minutes to indicate that the examiners should exchange roles. After 30 minutes a final bell will sound, the examiner will conclude the oral, and you may then leave the table.

Selection of Clinical Science oral questions

The format of the Clinical Science oral questions is similar regardless of the subject matter. The examiners are not looking for a list of regurgitated facts but wish to explore your understanding of basic medical scientific concepts in relation to clinical practice. The opening question will be clinical progressing to scientific principles.

Your Clinical Science oral will comprise four questions selected from the College question bank, a source of several hundred anatomy, physiology, pharmacology and clinical measurement oral questions. The examiners of the Clinical Science Oral Sub Group, who are responsible for selecting your questions, continually review, update and amend the question bank in response to examiner feedback, observer feedback, developments in anaesthetic practice and the performance of that question in previous examinations. The Clinical Science oral questions are also co-ordinated with the SAQ and the Clinical Oral questions in order to minimise duplication of specific subject areas in each sitting of the examination. All the candidates in the room will be asked the same four questions (although not necessarily in the same order) – one anatomy, one physiology, one pharmacology and one on physics/clinical measurement. Two of the questions will be asked by the first examiner and the remaining two by the second examiner. The time allocated to each question is approximately the same (~7.5 minutes) but there will be some flexibility exercised at the examiners' discretion. The examiners score each question independently.

Anatomy

A typical question would involve knowledge of the anatomy of the major organs, nerves or blood vessels relevant to surgery, acute and chronic pain management including neural blockade or practical procedures in theatres and intensive care. Maternal and fetal anatomy relevant to obstetric care, developmental anatomy after birth and anatomy of structures at risk of damage due to patient positioning are all included in the curriculum. Questions on the blood supply of the brain, heart or spinal cord, anatomy of the base of the skull or circulation of CSF regularly appear.

When preparing for the exam concentrate on the anatomy of structures that you can cannulate, block or intubate. Consider the surgical procedure being undertaken – what adjacent structures might be damaged and what complications occur? The anatomy curriculum is much more wide-ranging than questions on the brachial plexus, antecubital fossa and internal jugular vein. Recently a question on the oesophagus caused some consternation amongst candidates but it was entirely legitimate as we spend time inserting nasogastric tubes, temperature probes or doppler cardiac output monitors into it, the surgeons resect it and we anaesthetise for removal of foreign bodies from it.

Physiology

A comprehensive understanding of applied physiology is a prerequisite of safe clinical practice. The examiners will expect the candidate to demonstrate a level of understanding of applied physiology that supports this supposition. Aspects of applied physiology that are relevant to any area of clinical anaesthesia and the care of the critically ill can be explored. The wide-ranging curriculum is detailed by organ system in the CCT document and also includes the important topic of nutrition.

The difference between the Primary and Final approach to basic science examination can be illustrated by a recent question on blood glucose control. Primary would encompass textbook knowledge of blood glucose control mechanisms but the Final will test your knowledge on the additional areas of adverse outcomes related to blood glucose, evidence for the ideal or therapeutic level of glucose in the surgical or critical care patient, national guidelines or practical problems in blood glucose control.

Pharmacology

Candidates are expected to be familiar with the applied pharmacology of all commonly used drugs in the peri-operative care of the patient. This will include the practical application of pharmacodynamic and pharmacokinetic knowledge. The implications for anaesthesia and the interactions of concomitant prescription medication can be explored. The effects of the disease process on anaesthetic agents and drug handling, with particular reference to intensive care, acute and chronic pain management, should be understood. Alternatively, the pharmacology oral question can be a question on the principles of applied statistics and clinical trials as seen in the mainstream anaesthetic literature. Candidates should be familiar with the statistical fundamentals upon which most clinical research is based.

A recent question on total intravenous anaesthesia illustrates the scope of pharmacology questions within the clinical science SOE. A question on propofol included exploration of pharmacokinetic models for propofol and the concepts of effect site concentration and context-sensitive half-time but at least half the question was on the recommendations for safe clinical administration of TIVA and the possible causes of awareness.

Clinical Measurement

Candidates are expected to understand the basic scientific physical principles of anaesthetic equipment and of clinical measurement. The emphasis is on the clinical applications of clinical measurement, their value and limitations. It is worth, in your daily practice, asking yourself how any equipment, monitor or breathing system works. When you use a parameter such as blood pressure, intracranial pressure, cardiac output or end-tidal carbon dioxide to manage a patient revise how the value has been measured, the potential for error and how the information obtained guides management. Healthcare management may come into the question and the CCT document outlines the areas within this topic. For example, a question may start by asking the benefits of fluid administration in major surgery, go on to the techniques for measuring cardiac output and end with the principles whereby a lead clinician might evaluate new equipment that they are planning to purchase for their department.

General advice

It is imperative that you arrive in good time for your oral and relax as best you can. The examiners fully understand that you may feel anxious and nervous. Remember all of the examiners have been in the same position as you, some several times! This is your opportunity to convince the examiners that you are worthy of the Final FRCA.

The candidates who impress the examiners are those who do most of the talking and present their answers in an ordered, systematic, coherent and structured manner. This is unquestionably a skill that can only come from being confident of your own knowledge and with regular oral practice beforehand. The commonest mistake is failure to practise speaking aloud coherently in answer to a question – it is a different skill from providing written answers.

Listen carefully to the question. Answer the question that was asked, not the question you hoped for. If you do not understand the question, ask the examiner to repeat it or phrase it differently. If you get off to a bad start and wish to start again, say so. If you realise you have made a mistake then say so and offer your alternative answer. If the answer to a question is not immediately obvious to you, try talking it through from first principles. If a diagram helps you to answer a question, draw one. Consider your body language. Do not mumble behind your hands, talk too fast or too loudly. Avoid getting into a situation where your only answers are 'yes' or 'no' as the very reticent candidate is unlikely to pass the examination.

It can be very difficult for a candidate to judge how well they are performing in an oral examination. You may easily misjudge your performance and be convinced that you have failed. Remember that you do not have to get every single question correct to pass the SOE, indeed good examining technique is to establish the limit of your knowledge. Occasionally a very able candidate can successfully get through the structured questions quickly. The examiners may then choose to explore the candidate's depth and breadth of knowledge in more depth perhaps with a view to you being a potential prize winner.

Examination guidance

Dr Liam Brennan, Member of Council and Chairman, Final FRCA Examination

Candidates who are unsuccessful in either the written or oral component of the Final FRCA Examination more than once may request a guidance interview although this is no longer a mandatory requirement. Interviews are held at the College and various regional centres. Increasingly guidance interviews will be jointly co-ordinated by the College and Schools of Anaesthesia, with input from College examiners. This is because the College strongly believes that the issues that prevent candidates from being successful in the FRCA examinations must be considered in a local context and should involve input from the candidate's trainers and School officers.

In a locally conducted interview, the candidate meets with their local trainers and at least one current Final FRCA examiner. The interview is designed to help the candidate identify their problems with the examinations and suggest possible solutions. Everyone recognises that the interview may be very stressful for the candidate and everything is done to make the atmosphere as informal as possible. Remember this is not an examination! Besides the examiners and trainers the candidate may wish to ask their personal mentor, a friend or a family member to sit in on the interview as well.

The guidance interviews last around 30 minutes. It is relatively easy to say to a candidate, 'Work harder, practise and improve this area'. More demanding on everyone is to identify why the candidate has not already done this. This is where input from the local trainers and mentors can be very important. Until the candidate understands the level of knowledge and commitment required, and are prepared to give up almost all their spare time in the run-up to the exam, they will have difficulty in reaching the standard. There may be domestic or health-related problems that are preventing full engagement with exam preparation and it may be appropriate to air these issues.

A certain level of clinical experience is needed to pass the Final, but the examination focuses on principles and is aimed at an anaesthetist with roughly 18 months' experience at specialist registrar level. The examination focuses on the Intermediate Curriculum based around the major modules of training such as paediatrics, neuro, ICM, pain etc. Sitting the Final too early, particularly the SOEs, without gaining adequate exposure to the major modules is often a theme of candidates who attend for guidance. In addition, the examiners expect candidates to have a broad understanding of the scientific basis of anaesthesia and so remembering to refresh their knowledge of the Primary basic science curriculum is also a prerequisite to sitting the Final.

For a candidate to gain maximum benefit from the guidance interview it is helpful if they ensure that the pre-interview form is completed and that their College Tutor has made a brief assessment of the candidate's situation. The examiner will lead a discussion and will identify any themes that have contributed to the candidate's difficulties with the exam. At the end of the interview a summary of the discussion will be provided and agreed with the candidate. The summary may include advice on when the candidate should next sit the examination. A copy of the summary form will be sent to the College for audit purposes only.

Finally, guidance interviews are a resource to assist candidates who are struggling to pass the FRCA examinations. It is emphasised that they should be regarded as a means of maximising success in the future and not be used to dwell on performance and particularly their marks at previous attempts. If candidates feel aggrieved at how they were assessed in an examination, the College has review and appeal procedures which are available via the College website.

Appendix A: FRCA Examination changes

The majority of recent changes to the Final FRCA were introduced in September 2009, further changes were also introduced during 2010 and 2011.

Summary of changes recently applied to Final FRCA Exams

September 2008:

Final MCQs

Negative marking was removed from the Final FRCA MCQ Examinations.

September 2009:

Written Examinations

- The MCQ and Short Answer Questions (SAQ) examination marks are added together to give a single result. Both papers carry equal weight.
- The pass marks for each part of the examination are calculated in the current way.
- The pass mark for the combined examination, are the sum of the pass marks of the two papers.
- The written examination became stand-alone from the SOE examination, it is pass/fail and must be passed before applying to sit the SOE.
- A pass in the written examination is valid for two years.

Final SOE

- SOE 1 and SOE 2 were merged into a single SOE examination conducted in two sessions, each with two examiners, and with the number and content of the questions unchanged.
- The answer to each question is given a numerical score by each examiner.
- Each examiner independently marks every answer.
- The candidate's overall score is the total marks awarded by all the examiners for all the questions. Maximum score 40; pass mark 32.

September 2010:

Final MCQ

- The number of multiple true/false questions were reduced from 90 to 60.
- Thirty single best answer questions (SBA) were added to the paper.

Guidance

- No mandatory requirement for candidates to attend guidance interview.
- A candidate who repeatedly fails a component of the exam may request an interview.
- Interviews limited to one per examination part i.e. Primary or Final.
- Special consideration is no longer given in respect of refunds following guidance interviews. Non request/attendance of a guidance interview does not affect eligibility towards examinations.

March 2011:

Final written SAQ examination

- All questions marked out of 20 in accordance with the marking guides for each question, these are agreed at the appropriate Standard Setting Day. The Board of Examiners no longer awards 10% of the marks for each question for clarity, judgement and the ability to prioritise. Marks are no longer deducted for serious errors.

Change to be implemented in September 2012:

- With effect from 1st September 2012 the Final FRCA examination components will be open to any doctor practising anaesthesia in the NHS (subject to certain eligibility criteria).

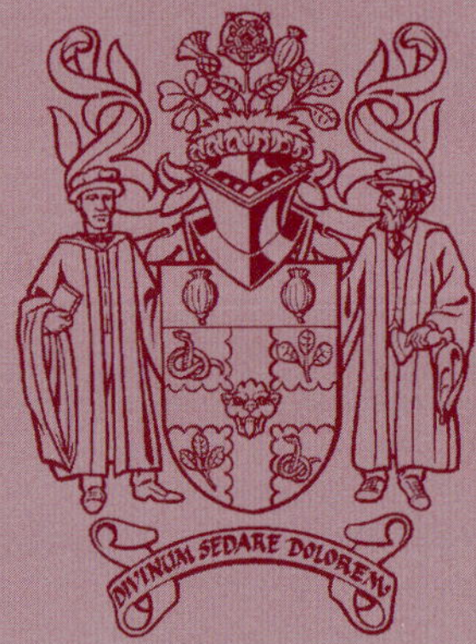
DIVINUM SEDARE DOLOREM

Section 2: Questions

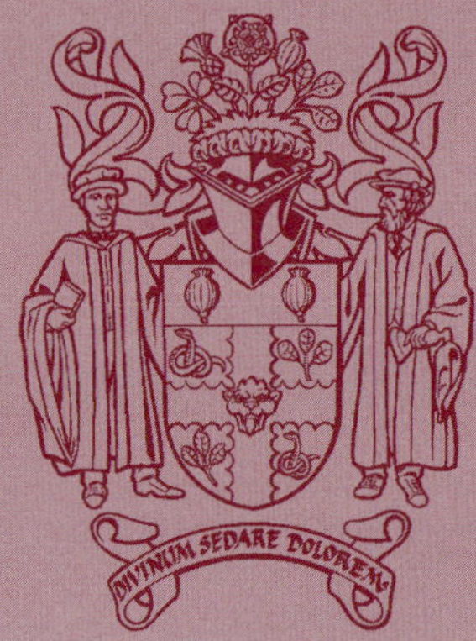
DIVINUM SEDARE DOLOREM

SAQ examination

SAQ Paper 1

Question 1

a List the advantages of day case surgical management compared with inpatient care. (30%)

b What are the surgical prerequisites that make a surgical procedure suitable for day case management? (30%)

c Summarise the discharge criteria that a patient needs to meet following a day case procedure. (40%)

Question 2

a Describe the type and course of primary pain afferents from the cornea to the brain. (20%)

b List the techniques which can provide local anaesthesia of the cornea. (20%)

c Which muscles and their innervations need to be blocked to achieve complete akinesia of the globe? (15%)

d What are the complications of sharp needle orbital blocks (30%) and how can they be minimised? (15%)

Question 3

What are the:

a cardiovascular (25%),

b respiratory (25%),

c gastrointestinal (20%), and

d haematological (30%) potential benefits of local anaesthetic neuraxial blockade?

Question 4

a Describe the initial management options following a paracetamol overdose. (25%)

b What clinical features may develop following an untreated paracetamol overdose? (45%)

c List the biochemical and haematological abnormalities that may occur at 72 hours following an untreated paracetamol overdose. (30%)

Question 5

A two-year-old child presents to the Emergency Department (ED) with sudden onset of fever (38.5°C aural), sore throat, drooling and stridor.

a What conditions should be considered in the differential diagnosis? (25%)

b What would be your initial management of this child in the ED? (30%)

c How would you subsequently manage a deteriorating child? (45%)

Question 6

a List the anaesthetic factors that predispose to peri-operative dental damage. (25%)

b List the patient-related factors that predispose to peri-operative dental damage. (25%)

c A 22-year-old man anaesthetised by a colleague awakens following tonsillectomy and complains that an upper incisor tooth has broken off during the operation. What is your management of this situation? (50%)

Question 7

a What are i) diagnostic and ii) other clinical features of severe pre-eclampsia? (40%)

b What are the indications for magnesium therapy in severe pre-eclampsia/eclampsia and which administration regimen(s) should be used? (20%)

c What are the symptoms and signs of magnesium toxicity (25%) and how should it be managed? (15%)

Question 8

a What are the considerations when administering a general anaesthetic to a patient in the neuroradiology suite? (50%)

b List the common interventional neuroradiological procedures that may require general anaesthesia. (25%)

c Outline the possible complications of interventional neuroradiological procedures. (25%)

Question 9

a List the effects of physiological or excess cortisol that are of anaesthetic relevance. (40%)

b What are the causes of adrenocortical insufficiency? (30%)

c How may acute corticosteroid insufficiency be diagnosed clinically and biochemically? (30%)

Question 10

a How may a patient with sickle cell disease present in an acute crisis? (20%)

b Outline the important pre-operative (30%), intra-operative (35%) and post-operative (15%) considerations when anaesthetising a patient with sickle cell disease for an elective procedure.

Question 11

a Define the term 'inadvertent peri-operative hypothermia'. (10%)

b What are the physical mechanisms by which heat is lost from a patient in an operating theatre? (25%)

c List the clinical complications of hypothermia in the peri-operative period. (30%)

d Outline the current recommendations in the UK for the prevention of peri-operative hypothermia. (35%)

Question 12

A 24-year-old male is scheduled for exploration and laying open of a pilonidal sinus under general anaesthesia.

a Outline the anaesthetic implications of managing this patient in the prone position. (45%)

b How may the complications of this position be minimised? (55%)

SAQ Paper 2

Question 1

a How may pain following Caesarean section (CS) performed under general anaesthesia be managed? (35%)

b What neuraxial techniques may be used to provide post-operative analgesia following CS? (Include appropriate dose ranges.) (20%)

c What are the monitoring requirements after CS following spinal or epidural opioid administration? (15%)

d List the side effects of neuraxially administered opioids, and how may these be managed? (30%)

Question 2

a What are the central and peripheral neurological complications of coronary artery bypass (CABG) surgery? (35%)

b What are the risk factors for central neurological complications following CABG surgery? (30%)

c How can the risk of central neurological complications of CABG surgery be reduced? (35%)

Question 3

A 67-year-old man requires a thoraco-abdominal oesophagectomy for adenocarcinoma.

a Describe the clinical features associated with the condition that are relevant to anaesthesia. (35%)

b List the pre-operative investigations you might need to consider. (30%)

c What aspects of peri-operative anaesthetic care can help reduce post-operative morbidity following this procedure? (35%)

Question 4

a Describe the anatomy of the cervical plexus. (40%)

b How would you perform a superficial cervical plexus block? (25%)

c A carotid endarterectomy is being performed using a superficial cervical plexus block. A few minutes after clamping the carotid artery the patient becomes unresponsive to verbal command. Describe your management of this situation. (35%)

Question 5

A 30-year-old man attempted suicide by jumping from a building. He sustained severe trauma including major facial injuries.

a What are the potential airway management problems? (25%)

b List five possible options for securing the airway in this patient. (25%)

c Outline the potential disadvantages for each of these options? (50%)

Question 6

a List the complications associated with the delivery of high partial pressures of oxygen? (60%)

b What are the oxygen saturation targets of oxygen therapy in: (i) previously healthy adult patients and (ii) patients with chronic obstructive pulmonary disease (COPD)? (10%)

c What are the postulated cellular mechanisms of oxygen toxicity? (10%)

d Which common themes associated with oxygen therapy were identified by the National Patient Safety Agency (NPSA) in 2009 as having contributed to patient deaths? (20%)

Question 7

a Describe the three essential stages of the World Health Organization (WHO) safety checklist, and when should they occur in relation to each operative procedure? (15%)

b What information needs to be exchanged between the anaesthetic, surgical and theatre teams as part of the checklist? (70%)

c Which aspects of the checklist are designed to decrease surgical site infection? (15%)

Question 8

a List the modes of non-invasive respiratory support (NIRS). (20%)

b In what adult clinical scenarios may NIRS be indicated? (30%)

c What are the contraindications to NIRS? (30%)

d Summarise the clinical advantages of NIRS compared to conventional positive pressure ventilation via a tracheal tube. (20%)

Question 9

a List the harmful chemicals in tobacco smoke. (15%)

b What are the pathophysiological effects of tobacco smoking on the cardiovascular (20%), respiratory (25%) and other body systems? (20%)

c What advice would you give to a smoker attending a pre-operative assessment clinic six weeks before a scheduled procedure under general anaesthesia? (20%)

Question 10

a What are the potential benefits of an enhanced recovery ('fast-track') programme for a patient undergoing major abdominal surgery? (25%)

b List the pre-operative (25%), intra-operative (25%) and post-operative goals (25%) that aim to achieve 'fast track' status.

Question 11

a What are the diagnostic (25%) and therapeutic (25%) indications for bronchoscopy?

b List the major contraindications for bronchoscopy. (20%)

c How should a fibreoptic bronchoscope be reprocessed after use? (30%)

Question 12

You are asked to assess a 4-year-old child who is scheduled for a strabismus (squint) correction as a day case procedure.

a List the anaesthetic-related issues this case presents. (60%)

b During surgical traction, the patient suddenly develops a profound sinus bradycardia. How would you manage this situation? (10%)

c Describe the key post-operative problems and relevant management strategies. (30%)

MCQ examination Multiple True or False (MTF)

1 **The following are indications for pre-operative measurement of serum urea and electrolytes in patients admitted for elective surgery:**

- **a** digoxin therapy
- **b** well controlled insulin dependent diabetes
- **c** recurrent urinary tract infections
- **d** diuretic therapy
- **e** all patients over fifty years old

2 **Hazards of anaesthesia in a patient with chronic renal failure include:**

- **a** left ventricular enlargement
- **b** pericarditis
- **c** hypertension
- **d** enhanced carotid sinus activity
- **e** cardiac tamponade

3 **Hypophysectomy may result in:**

- **a** atrophy of the thyroid
- **b** osteoporosis
- **c** atrophy of the adrenal cortex
- **d** diabetes insipidus
- **e** diabetes mellitus

4 **The following groups of people have an increased risk of latex allergy:**

- **a** healthcare workers
- **b** those with penicillin allergy
- **c** those with fruit allergy
- **d** those who have had repeated tracheal intubation
- **e** those who have had repeated surgical procedures

5 **Myocardial stunning:**

- **a** is irreversible
- **b** always follows myocardial ischaemia
- **c** is appropriately treated using dobutamine
- **d** causes beta adrenoceptor down-regulation
- **e** is reduced by cardioplegia solution

6 **Supraclavicular brachial plexus block differs from axillary brachial plexus block because the supraclavicular block:**

- **a** gives a lower incidence of analgesia for the lateral part of the forearm
- **b** is less likely to involve nerves to the intraosseous muscles
- **c** produces analgesia of the shoulder joint
- **d** is more likely to cause pneumothorax
- **e** is more likely to involve an intravascular injection of local anaesthetic

7 **Severe middle third fractures of the face:**

- **a** are associated with brain injury
- **b** cause breathing difficulties
- **c** always require immediate fixation
- **d** require the patient to be intubated through the nose for fixation
- **e** include fractures of the orbit and zygoma

8 **Phantom limb pain:**

- **a** is more common if there was pain in the limb before amputation
- **b** is effectively treated by sympathetic block
- **c** is treated by ablation of the relevant motor nerves
- **d** is treated by transcutaneous electrical nerve stimulation
- **e** is not a feature of traumatic amputation of a limb

9 **Pain during the first stage of labour may be relieved by:**

- **a** epidural block
- **b** spinal block
- **c** pudendal nerve block
- **d** paracervical block
- **e** lumbar sympathetic block

10 **Symptoms or signs characteristic of amniotic fluid embolism include:**

- **a** cyanosis
- **b** hypofibrinogenaemia
- **c** chest pain
- **d** hypoventilation
- **e** hypertension

11 **At a core temperature of 30°C:**

- **a** oxygen consumption is reduced to approximately 50% of that at 37°C
- **b** blood coagulability is increased
- **c** glomerular filtration ceases
- **d** blood viscosity is reduced
- **e** the solubility of carbon dioxide in the blood is increased

12 In a patient with porphyria:

- **a** etomidate may produce an acute attack
- **b** glycine should not be used in irrigating solutions during trans-urethral resection (TUR) of the prostate
- **c** dysautonomia may be present
- **d** pre-operative fluid restriction protects against an acute attack intra-operatively
- **e** fentanyl may be used safely

13 In myotonic dystrophy, spasticity of muscles is relieved by:

- **a** succinylcholine
- **b** spinal anaesthesia
- **c** neostigmine
- **d** infiltration of the muscle with lidocaine
- **e** dantrolene

14 Cardioversion is indicated in the treatment of:

- **a** sinus tachycardia
- **b** atrial flutter
- **c** junctional bradycardia
- **d** ventricular tachycardia
- **e** electro-mechanical dissociation

15 Circulatory assistance by intra-aortic balloon pumping is useful because it:

- **a** increases aortic diastolic pressure
- **b** increases aortic systolic pressure
- **c** decreases myocardial oxygen demand
- **d** increases left atrial pressure
- **e** increases left ventricular end-diastolic pressure

16 **During storage of whole blood, the decrease in 2,3-diphosphoglycerate (2,3-DPG) concentration can be reduced by the addition of:**

- **a** mannitol
- **b** adenosine
- **c** pyruvate
- **d** phosphate
- **e** glucose

17 **In a sacral epidural (caudal) block in adults:**

- **a** the sacral hiatus can be located by reference to the posterior superior iliac spines
- **b** the lower extremity of the dura is normally 3–4 cm below the level of the posterior superior iliac spines
- **c** the sacral canal can be identified using a technique based on the negative pressure in the canal
- **d** absorption of local anaesthetic is greater than from the lumbar epidural space
- **e** a subcutaneous malposition of the needle can be confirmed by injecting air

18 **Structures supplied by segment S2 include the:**

- **a** skin of the buttock
- **b** skin of the back of the leg
- **c** bladder
- **d** flexor hallucis longus
- **e** gluteus maximus

19 **Interruption of the cervical sympathetic chain results in:**

- **a** dilatation of the pupil on the affected side
- **b** loss of taste sensation over the anterior two-thirds of the tongue
- **c** partial ptosis on the same side
- **d** dryness of the mouth
- **e** absence of thermal sweating on the same side of the face

20 The following agents may cause pulmonary fibrosis:

- [ ] **a** bleomycin
- [ ] **b** cortisone hemisuccinate
- [ ] **c** beryllium
- [ ] **d** paraquat
- [ ] **e** organophosphate compounds

21 Heat and moisture exchange filters:

- [ ] **a** should have a high thermal capacity
- [ ] **b** become more efficient as tidal volume and minute volume are increased
- [ ] **c** should have a low thermal conductivity for maximum efficiency
- [ ] **d** should have a resistance of less than 5 cm H_2O L^{-1} sec^{-1} after 24 hours simulated use
- [ ] **e** should filter out particles of greater than two micrometres diameter

22 An abnormal response to suxamethonium occurs in patients suffering from:

- [ ] **a** polyarteritis nodosa
- [ ] **b** dermatomyositis
- [ ] **c** systemic lupus erythematosus
- [ ] **d** dystrophia myotonica
- [ ] **e** hepatic failure

23 The ventilatory response to hypoxia is decreased in patients:

- [ ] **a** with cyanotic congenital heart disease
- [ ] **b** emerging from isoflurane anaesthesia
- [ ] **c** with chronic exposure to high altitude
- [ ] **d** with pulmonary fibrosis
- [ ] **e** on a patient-demand opiate infusion

24 **The following drugs alter the level of thyroxine production:**

- **a** amiodarone
- **b** propylthiouracil
- **c** propranolol
- **d** carbidopa
- **e** prazocin

25 **Stimulation of postganglionic thoraco-lumbar autonomic nerve fibres produces:**

- **a** cutaneous vasoconstriction
- **b** bronchiolar constriction
- **c** secretion of eccrine sweat glands
- **d** a reduction in myocardial rhythmicity
- **e** a reduction in myocardial contractility

26 **The alveolar-arterial oxygen tension difference is increased by:**

- **a** a high inspired oxygen concentration
- **b** nitrous oxide uptake
- **c** a reduction in functional residual capacity
- **d** an increase in ventilation/perfusion mismatch
- **e** hepatic failure

27 **Pulmonary vascular resistance is reduced by:**

- **a** hypoxia
- **b** hypercarbia
- **c** alkalosis
- **d** epoprostenol (prostacyclin)
- **e** nitric oxide

28 **Complement is required for:**

- **a** clearance of both endotoxin and bacteraemia
- **b** apoptosis
- **c** normal C reactive protein release
- **d** membrane attack complex
- **e** normal activation of the coagulation cascade

29 **Clonidine:**

- **a** inhibits alpha-2 adrenoceptors
- **b** cannot cross the blood brain barrier
- **c** reduces heart rate
- **d** has analgesic properties
- **e** is a respiratory stimulant

30 **Xenon:**

- **a** has a MAC value of approximately 70% in oxygen
- **b** acts preferentially at the N-methyl-D-aspartate (NMDA) receptor
- **c** can be measured by changes in the refractive index of light
- **d** is more soluble in blood than sevoflurane
- **e** produces analgesia when inhaled as a 50% mixture with oxygen

31 **In determining the pulmonary shunt fraction (Qs/Qt), which of the following information is required:**

- **a** FiO_2
- **b** mixed venous oxygen content
- **c** cardiac output
- **d** P_aCO_2
- **e** arterial oxygen content

32 **The recurrent laryngeal nerve innervates the:**

- **a** cricothyroid muscle
- **b** posterior cricoarytenoid muscle
- **c** mucous membrane of the trachea
- **d** thyrohyoid muscle
- **e** vocalis muscle

33 **The sacral canal contains:**

- **a** no cerebrospinal fluid
- **b** less than 10 ml of injected local anaesthetic
- **c** roots of the sciatic nerve
- **d** roots of the genitofemoral nerve
- **e** roots of the ilioinguinal nerve

34 **A drug which blocks dopamine receptors only is likely to:**

- **a** delay gastric emptying
- **b** reduce renal perfusion
- **c** be effective in motion sickness
- **d** be useful in treating Parkinsonism
- **e** have anti-arrhythmic properties

35 **These drugs selectively increase renal blood flow:**

- **a** dobutamine
- **b** dopamine
- **c** dopexamine
- **d** digoxin
- **e** diazoxide

36 **The following factors enhance the diffusion of a drug across the blood brain barrier:**

- **a** high lipid-solubility
- **b** high plasma protein binding
- **c** high plasma-brain concentration gradient
- **d** high degree of ionisation at physiological pH
- **e** high molecular weight

37 **Sevoflurane:**

- **a** has a boiling point of 50.2°C
- **b** has a blood/gas partition coefficient of 0.46
- **c** must be protected from light during storage
- **d** is degraded in the body with the production of fluoride ions
- **e** is a molecule which contains a chlorine atom

38 **Intraocular pressure is lowered by:**

- **a** hypocapnoea
- **b** isoflurane
- **c** hypoxia
- **d** propofol
- **e** non-depolarising neuromuscular blocking drugs

39 **Appropriate nerve blocks for the treatment of pain associated with chronic pancreatitis include:**

- **a** lumbar sympathetic
- **b** thoracic paravertebral
- **c** coeliac plexus
- **d** thoracic extradural
- **e** intrathecal phenol

40 **Causes of low arterial pressure upon initiation of cardiopulmonary bypass with total crystalloid prime include:**

- **a** inadequate venous return
- **b** low haematocrit
- **c** low viscosity
- **d** hypothermia
- **e** inadequate oxygen carriage

41 **Surgical closure of a patent ductus arteriosus produces:**

- **a** obliteration of the murmur
- **b** increased oxygenation of blood
- **c** increased diastolic pressure
- **d** decreased pulmonary artery pressure
- **e** decreased left ventricular output

42 **Emergency treatment of severe hypotension unresponsive to ephedrine in a fit patient undergoing cervical laminectomy in the sitting position includes:**

- **a** turning the patient on to the right side
- **b** intra-aortic balloon counterpulsation
- **c** intravenous administration of $NaHCO_3$
- **d** placing the patient in the head down position
- **e** withdrawing nitrous oxide

43 **Paraplegic patients with spinal cord transection at T6 for more than one year manifest:**

- **a** a labile arterial blood pressure
- **b** mass autonomic reflex
- **c** hyperkalaemia after intravenous succinylcholine
- **d** hypoventilation
- **e** causalgia

44 For laryngoscopy:

- a the ideal position for the head involves extension of the cervical spine
- b a polio Macintosh blade for difficult intubation is mounted at 180° to the handle
- c the Macintosh 3 blade is available in a left-handed version
- d the light emitted from a fibreoptic laryngoscope blade deteriorates when autoclaved
- e previous surgery for a thyroglossal cyst will make laryngoscopy with a Macintosh blade easier

45 Complications of deep cervical plexus block include:

- a Bell's palsy
- b hoarseness
- c bradycardia
- d dyspnoea
- e ipsilateral mydriasis

46 Inadvertent surgical stimulation of the fifth cranial nerve during posterior fossa craniotomy will produce:

- a jerking of the jaw
- b facial twitching
- c bradycardia
- d jerking of the shoulder
- e nystagmus

47 The hypertensive response to laryngoscopy and tracheal intubation may be attenuated by:

- a enalapril
- b buprenorphine
- c lidocaine spray to the cords and trachea
- d glycopyrrolate
- e intravenous lidocaine

48 **Appropriate recommendations for the peri-operative management of an Afro-Caribbean child scheduled for urgent internal fixation of a closed tibial fracture, whose haemoglobin is found to be 7.5 g dl^{-1} despite minimal blood loss, include:**

- **a** postponing the operation until haemoglobin electrophoresis is available
- **b** pre-operative administration of packed cells until the haemoglobin is 10 g dl^{-1}
- **c** administration of parenteral hydrocortisone and proceeding with the operation
- **d** using hypotensive anaesthesia to avoid transfusion
- **e** avoiding succinylcholine in a rapid sequence induction

49 **Appropriate management of a female patient with untreated thyrotoxicosis requiring repair of an incarcerated femoral hernia includes:**

- **a** intravenous propranolol
- **b** atropine premedication
- **c** spinal anaesthesia
- **d** intravenous chlorpromazine
- **e** intravenous carbimazole

50 **In assessing the adequacy of medullary perfusion during posterior fossa surgery, the appearance of the following are useful:**

- **a** delta waves in the electroencephalogram
- **b** hypothermia
- **c** increase in mean arterial blood pressure
- **d** cardiac arrhythmia
- **e** irregularities in respiration

51 **During general anaesthesia for laparoscopy when the intra-abdominal pressure is 40 mmHg the following parameters would decrease:**

- **a** central venous pressure
- **b** heart rate
- **c** cardiac output
- **d** systemic vascular resistance
- **e** airway pressure

52 **A continuous positive pressure breathing system (CPAP) for an adult:**

- **a** requires a fresh gas flow of 15 L min^{-1}
- **b** improves oxygenation in patients by an increase in functional residual capacity
- **c** should maintain pressure during inspiration within 0.5 kPa (5 cm H_2O) of the pressure during expiration
- **d** if used correctly will reduce lung compliance
- **e** may increase the work of breathing

53 **When performing the 'three-in-one' block for pain relief in lower limb surgery:**

- **a** the needle is inserted medial to the femoral artery
- **b** the saphenous nerve will be blocked
- **c** good analgesia will be obtained for operations on the foot
- **d** the obturator nerve, femoral nerve and the lateral cutaneous nerve of the thigh will be blocked
- **e** muscle relaxation is provided

54 **The hazard of microshock in hospital can be reduced by use of:**

- **a** isolated (floating) power supply
- **b** saline-filled intracardiac catheters
- **c** battery powered appliances
- **d** multiple earth paths
- **e** large area diathermy plates

55 **Malignant hyperthermia:**

- **a** is associated with Duchenne muscular dystrophy
- **b** may be precipitated by stress
- **c** is inherited as an autosomal recessive
- **d** is more frequent in males
- **e** has an incidence of approximately 1 in 15,000 children

56 **A neurolytic coeliac plexus block:**

- **a** causes postural hypotension
- **b** is performed anterolateral to the body of L2
- **c** causes neuropathic pain in the upper thigh
- **d** causes diarrhoea
- **e** is performed with the needle placed anterior to the aorta

57 **Surgical correction of scoliosis:**

- **a** carries a high risk of spinal cord damage
- **b** is monitored by somatosensory evoked potentials
- **c** is facilitated by induced hypotension
- **d** may involve division of the diaphragm
- **e** typically requires post-operative ventilation for several days

58 **After successful supraclavicular brachial plexus block, sensory anaesthesia will usually be incomplete on the:**

- **a** medial aspect of the forearm
- **b** lateral aspect of the forearm
- **c** lateral aspect of the upper arm
- **d** medial aspect of the upper arm
- **e** back of the elbow

59 **Retro-bulbar block:**

- **a** dilates the pupils
- **b** causes enophthalmos
- **c** reduces intraocular pressure
- **d** prevents lachrymation
- **e** increases the likelihood of vitreous prolapse

60 **Premature neonates:**

- **a** are prone to develop hypocalcaemia
- **b** are sensitive to non-depolarising relaxants
- **c** have reduced insensible water loss
- **d** have increased unconjugated bilirubin levels
- **e** have excess Type 1 (oxidative) muscle fibres in the diaphragm

61 **The TURP syndrome:**

- **a** is associated with hypokalaemia
- **b** may present with convulsions
- **c** is prevented by spinal anaesthesia
- **d** is due to blood loss
- **e** requires a diuretic for its treatment

62 **The group A antigen:**

- **a** is carried by all the red blood cells of a group A patient
- **b** is the most common cause of haemolytic disease of the newborn
- **c** can occur in the saliva of a group A patient
- **d** is transmitted according to Mendelian principles
- **e** is more common than group B antigen in Caucasians

63 **The penicillins:**

- **a** are bacteriostatic
- **b** interfere with bacterial cell wall synthesis
- **c** are more active against organisms which are not dividing
- **d** do not affect Gram-positive cocci
- **e** are all destroyed by penicillinase

64 **The following are competitive antagonists:**

- **a** neostigmine
- **b** naltrexone
- **c** buprenorphine
- **d** flumazenil
- **e** enoximone

65 **Intra-operative signs of a haemolytic transfusion reaction include:**

- **a** an increase in capillary bleeding
- **b** hypertension
- **c** fever
- **d** urticaria
- **e** periorbital oedema

66 **Dopamine:**

- **a** demonstrates a renal protective effect
- **b** increases intracellular calcium concentration
- **c** usually increases cardiac output at 2 $\mu g\ kg^{-1}\ min^{-1}$
- **d** increases creatinine clearance
- **e** increases splanchnic oxygen requirement

67 **Lactic acid is:**

] **a** formed during anaerobic ATP re-synthesis
] **b** increased in concentration in the blood during energy deficit
] **c** not formed by red blood cells
] **d** converted to glucose by the Cori cycle
] **e** oxidised without conversion back to glucose

68 **Low molecular weight heparin:**

] **a** activity is effectively measured by APTT
] **b** has a longer plasma half-life than standard heparin
] **c** strongly binds to plasma proteins
] **d** has its effect completely reversed by an equivalent dose of protamine
] **e** has prolonged plasma clearance in patients with renal failure

69 **The blood brain barrier:**

] **a** is composed mainly of endothelial cells
] **b** restricts passive diffusion of glucose from blood to brain
] **c** is functionally affected by CNS infection
] **d** is less permeable in neonates than adults
] **e** restricts passive diffusion of lipophilic drugs from blood to brain

70 **In normal individuals with a normal P_aCO_2, cerebral blood flow:**

] **a** autoregulates between cerebral perfusion pressures of 50–100 mmHg
] **b** is reduced when breathing 100% oxygen
] **c** increases with hypothermia
] **d** is normally 45 ml 100 g^{-1} min^{-1}
] **e** increases following the administration of mannitol 0.5 g kg^{-1}

71 **In normal pregnancy:**

- **a** the plasma colloid osmotic pressure decreases to about 17 mmHg
- **b** the total quantity of plasma proteins is decreased
- **c** the concentration of most globulins increases
- **d** altered plasma protein levels increase the toxicity of bupivacaine
- **e** plasma volume increases to 60 ml kg^{-1}

72 **The alpha-2 adrenoreceptor agonist clonidine:**

- **a** reduces the dose requirement for inhalational anaesthetics
- **b** increases heart rate
- **c** reduces arterial blood pressure
- **d** antagonises the analgesic effect of opioids
- **e** increases the duration of epidurally administered bupivacaine

73 **Intercostal nerves:**

- **a** pass anterior to the posterior intercostal membrane
- **b** pass between the external and internal intercostal muscles
- **c** lie superior to the intercostal artery and vein
- **d** give rise to lateral and anterior cutaneous branches
- **e** supply the periphery of the diaphragm

74 **Pulmonary vascular resistance is:**

- **a** increased if the haematocrit is abnormally high
- **b** decreased when breathing 79% helium with 21% oxygen
- **c** increased by the application of 5 cm H_2O positive end-expiratory pressure
- **d** increased by breathing 2% sevoflurane in air
- **e** decreased by moderate exercise

75 **The following are nephrotoxic:**

- **a** angiotensin converting enzyme inhibitors
- **b** non-steroidal anti-inflammatory drugs
- **c** halothane
- **d** aminoglycosides
- **e** radiocontrast agents

76 **Shock due to Gram-negative bacteraemia is frequently associated with:**

- **a** oliguria
- **b** hypotension unresponsive to fluid replacement
- **c** pre-existing jaundice
- **d** intermittent fever
- **e** low cardiac output

77 **After a severe burn (greater than 40% full thickness):**

- **a** enteral nutrition should be started as soon as possible
- **b** vascular access should never be placed through burned skin
- **c** fluid requirements are maximal in the first 12 hours
- **d** tissue swelling is maximal between 24 and 48 hours
- **e** prophylactic antibiotics should be given

78 **In the critically ill, skeletal muscle:**

- **a** has decreased free intracellular glutamine
- **b** demonstrates decreased muscle protein synthesis
- **c** breakdown can be prevented by early nutritional support
- **d** breakdown is prevented by endogenous cortisol
- **e** shows an increased myofibrillar protein synthesis when insulin is administered

79 **The use of propofol for sedation on the Intensive Care Unit is associated with:**

- **a** a calorie load of 0.1 kcal ml^{-1}
- **b** raised serum triglycerides
- **c** increased cerebral blood flow
- **d** a reduction in mean arterial pressure
- **e** reduced shunt

80 **Mixed venous oxygen saturation is:**

- **a** increased in anaemia
- **b** increased in hypothermia
- **c** decreased when cardiac output is low
- **d** decreased in established systemic sepsis
- **e** can be measured continuously using fibreoptics

81 **The crush syndrome:**

- **a** results from extensive tissue ischaemia
- **b** results in myoglobinuria
- **c** renal damage is more likely if the urine is acidic
- **d** commonly causes disseminated intravascular coagulation
- **e** is seen in compartment syndromes

82 **Important measures to prevent hospital acquired infections in intensive care include:**

- **a** adequate separation of beds as specified in national standards
- **b** separation of new admissions from the rest of the intensive care patients
- **c** plastic overshoes
- **d** routine culture of the environment and equipment
- **e** changing ventilator tubing every 24 hours

83 **Potential complications of the use of neuromuscular blocking agents in the critically ill include:**

- **a** venous thromboembolism
- **b** critical illness neuropathy
- **c** cardiac arrhythmias
- **d** protracted muscle weakness
- **e** peripheral nerve injury

84 **Electrocardiographic changes during hypothermia to 28°C include:**

- **a** ventricular extrasystole
- **b** peaked T waves
- **c** atrial fibrillation
- **d** left bundle branch block
- **e** bigeminy

85 **Ionised calcium:**

- **a** may be measured in a sodium-heparin (blood gas) sample
- **b** is measured in a 'clotted' (serum) specimen
- **c** is affected by pH
- **d** falls during massive blood transfusion
- **e** is affected by changes in serum proteins

86 **In thermal dilution techniques for the measurement of cardiac output:**

- **a** the bolus of injectate should have a volume of at least 20 ml
- **b** it is necessary to obtain a reading of wedge pressure
- **c** the result is inaccurate if the patient is febrile
- **d** the bolus should be injected rapidly
- **e** the result is unaffected by the phase of the respiratory cycle in which the injection is made

87 **A typical daily regimen for total parenteral nutrition in an adult:**

- a includes 14 g nitrogen per day
- b should avoid fat emulsions in patients with liver failure
- c includes glucose
- d includes magnesium
- e includes approximately 1 ml water for each kilocalorie given

88 **The effectiveness of defibrillation is increased by:**

- a delivery during inspiration
- b acidosis
- c pretreatment with class 1a anti-arrhythmics
- d amiodarone
- e ensuring uniform distribution of applied current within the heart

89 **Signs of overdose of a tricyclic antidepressant include:**

- a tachycardia
- b meiosis
- c urinary retention
- d myocardial depression
- e flushed dry skin

90 **In the following situations the measured pulmonary artery occlusion pressure (PAOP) will not reflect left ventricular end-diastolic pressure (LVEDP):**

- a catheter placement in West zone III
- b mitral incompetence
- c tricuspid incompetence
- d pulmonary embolus
- e aortic stenosis

91 Hypophosphataemia gives rise to:

- **a** difficulty in weaning patients from a ventilator
- **b** shift of the oxygen dissociation curve to the right
- **c** increased red cell fragility
- **d** reversible myocardial dysfunction
- **e** a peripheral neuropathy

92 The following are endogenous pro-inflammatory cytokines:

- **a** tumour necrosis factor alpha
- **b** interleukin 6
- **c** interleukin 1ra
- **d** interleukin 10
- **e** nuclear factor kappa B

93 The treatment of amitriptyline poisoning includes:

- **a** forced diuresis
- **b** an isoprenaline infusion
- **c** digitalisation
- **d** intravenous atropine sulphate
- **e** beta adrenoceptor antagonists

94 Conditions associated with smoke inhalation injury include:

- **a** the immediate development of pulmonary oedema
- **b** sloughing of the mucosa of the upper airway
- **c** a shift of the oxyhaemoglobin dissociation curve to the left
- **d** heat injury to the lung parenchyma
- **e** increased carboxyhaemoglobin concentration

95 **Nosocomial pneumonia is:**

- **a** the most common hospital acquired infection
- **b** associated with a high reported mortality rate (20–50%)
- **c** most often due to Enterobacteriaceae
- **d** minimised by hand washing
- **e** associated with the use of H_2 blockers in hospital patients

96 **Likely causes of severe hypotension following surgical removal of a phaeochromocytoma include:**

- **a** inadequate pre-operative alpha adrenoceptor blockade
- **b** acute adrenal cortical failure
- **c** hypersensitive beta receptors
- **d** diminished plasma volume
- **e** splanchnic pooling

97 **Criteria applied in the diagnosis of 'brain death' include:**

- **a** absence of activity in any cranial nerve
- **b** fixed non-reactive pupils
- **c** absent doll's eye reflex
- **d** upgoing plantar reflexes
- **e** two 'flat' EEG tracings repeated 24 hours apart

98 **The effects of Ecstasy (3,4-methylenedioxymethamphetamine):**

- **a** are usually dose-related
- **b** include hyperpyrexia, hypercalcaemia, and hyperkalaemia
- **c** are due to inhibition of 5-hydroxytryptamine
- **d** are due to drinking large amounts of water
- **e** include renal failure due to rhabdomyolysis

99 **Endotoxin:**

] **a** is detected in over 70% of patients suffering from sepsis syndrome
] **b** may be degraded by administered antibodies directed to the O antigen
] **c** can be detected with a test using crab blood
] **d** if injected into volunteers lowers pulmonary arterial pressure
] **e** consists of two main components

100 **In acute hepatic failure:**

] **a** the prothrombin time is in excess of 20 seconds
] **b** serum alkaline phosphatase may be normal
] **c** serum albumin levels are usually normal
] **d** plasma bilirubin is a sensitive indicator of hepatocellular damage
] **e** serum LDH is a sensitive index of hepatocellular damage

101 **In children, death from severe burns in the second week after injury is likely to be due to:**

] **a** haemoconcentration
] **b** anaemia
] **c** toxaemia from protein destruction
] **d** hepatic failure
] **e** infection of the burned area

102 **The risk of infection in a central venous catheter:**

] **a** is greater with the internal jugular than the subclavian approach
] **b** is greater with triple lumen than single lumen catheters
] **c** depends on catheter material
] **d** is minimised by the use of an occlusive transparent plastic dressing
] **e** is minimised by the use of a cut down surgical technique

103 A rapid shallow breathing pattern in the critically ill:

- a is seen in patients in acute respiratory failure
- b is associated with failure to wean from ventilation
- c results from a high P_aCO_2
- d is due to hypoxaemia
- e almost always reflects respiratory muscle weakness

104 Fluoroquinolones:

- a are chemically related to nalidixic acid
- b are effective against pneumococci
- c are effective in Gram-negative pneumonia
- d may cause seizures
- e are chelated by aluminium salts

105 The following measurements are consistent with physiological oliguria:

- a urine sodium < 10 mmol L^{-1}
- b urine specific gravity > 1.024
- c urine/plasma osmolality ratio 5:1
- d urine/plasma urea 100:1
- e urine/plasma creatinine 20:1

106 Side effects of amiodarone include:

- a peripheral neuropathy
- b hypothyroidism
- c corneal microdeposits
- d photosensitisation
- e bigeminal rhythm

107 Patients at greater than normal risk of developing Gram-negative bacteraemia include those suffering from:

- **a** diabetes mellitus
- **b** cirrhosis
- **c** leukaemia
- **d** polycythaemia
- **e** uraemia

108 In a patient suffering from paroxysmal nocturnal dyspnoea the following signs would favour asthma rather than left ventricular failure:

- **a** raised jugular venous pressure
- **b** basal crepitations
- **c** expiratory wheeze in the absence of other signs
- **d** central cyanosis early in the attack
- **e** hypotension

109 Trans-oesophageal echocardiography:

- **a** can be used to measure intraventricular pressure changes
- **b** is useful for observing tricuspid regurgitation
- **c** can give an index of stroke volume
- **d** is helpful in assessing myocardial ischaemia
- **e** is helpful in assessing myocardial contractility

110 Morbid obesity:

- **a** results in a lower blood volume on a volume per weight basis
- **b** decreases oxygen flux
- **c** reduces hypoxic pulmonary vasoconstriction
- **d** can result in left axis deviation on the ECG
- **e** causes insulin resistance

111 **In an otherwise normal person, chronic iron deficiency anaemia with a haemoglobin concentration of 60 g/L is associated with:**

- **a** metabolic acidosis
- **b** decreased right atrial PO_2
- **c** decreased left atrial PO_2
- **d** increased heart rate
- **e** shift of the oxyhaemoglobin curve to the left

112 **The pulmonary artery wedge pressure is a good indicator of left ventricular end-diastolic pressure in patients suffering from:**

- **a** myocardial infarction
- **b** mitral stenosis
- **c** aortic stenosis
- **d** pulmonary stenosis
- **e** cardiomyopathy

113 **The development of high titres of anti D antibodies in a Rhesus negative mother with an Rh positive fetus:**

- **a** is due to fetal red blood cells entering the maternal circulation
- **b** will result in anaemia of the newborn
- **c** will result in jaundice of the newborn
- **d** is due to antigen alone entering the maternal circulation
- **e** always occurs before the third month of gestation

114 **An acutely developing blood coagulation defect associated with massive transfusion may be due to:**

- **a** thrombocytopenia
- **b** disseminated intravascular coagulation
- **c** deficiency of clotting Factors V and VIII
- **d** incompatible transfusion reaction
- **e** fibrinolysis

115 Platelet concentrate:

- **a** remains viable for two weeks
- **b** is stored at 4°C
- **c** contains citrate
- **d** requires cross-matching
- **e** significantly elevates plasma histamine concentrations

116 In pulmonary contusion there will be:

- **a** crepitations on auscultation
- **b** radiological evidence of pulmonary opacity within six hours of blunt chest trauma
- **c** blood tinged tracheal secretions
- **d** an increased alveolar–arterial oxygen tension gradient
- **e** increased lung compliance

117 Recognised complications of bronchial neoplasms include:

- **a** hypercalcaemia
- **b** hyperkalaemia
- **c** inappropriate ADH secretion
- **d** Cushing's syndrome
- **e** hypothyroidism

118 The following symptoms strongly suggest a diagnosis of transient cerebral ischaemia:

- **a** monocular visual loss of two-hour duration
- **b** transient global amnesia
- **c** deafness
- **d** dysphasia that almost resolves by 72 hours
- **e** three episodes of dysarthria, each of which recovers completely within six hours

119 **A history of alcoholism is associated with:**

- **a** malnutrition
- **b** increased adrenocortical response to surgery
- **c** delayed gastric emptying
- **d** an MCV of 95 fl
- **e** a raised plasma albumin level

120 **Effects of hypermagnesaemia include:**

- **a** inhibition of acetylcholine release at the neuromuscular junction
- **b** decreased sensitivity of the motor end-plate to acetylcholine
- **c** augmented action of succinylcholine
- **d** reduced action of pancuronium
- **e** decreased myocardial contractility

121 **Bilateral hilar lymphadenopathy is a feature of:**

- **a** pulmonary tuberculosis
- **b** Hodgkin's disease
- **c** erythema multiforme
- **d** pneumoconiosis
- **e** systemic lupus erythematosus

122 **A low fixed cardiac output is associated with:**

- **a** aortic stenosis
- **b** constrictive pericarditis
- **c** mitral stenosis
- **d** cor pulmonale
- **e** digoxin toxicity

123 Collapse of the lower lobe of the right lung is characterised by:

- [ ] **a** an increased alveolar–arterial oxygen tension difference
- [ ] **b** an increased P_aCO_2
- [ ] **c** an area of stony dullness to percussion
- [ ] **d** a decreased arterial pH
- [ ] **e** tachypnoea

124 A haemoglobin of 8 g dl^{-1} with a reticulocyte count of 10% is associated with:

- [ ] **a** aplastic anaemia
- [ ] **b** untreated pernicious anaemia
- [ ] **c** polycythaemia
- [ ] **d** haemolytic anaemia
- [ ] **e** acute leukaemia

125 Causes of atrial fibrillation include:

- [ ] **a** thyrotoxicosis
- [ ] **b** rheumatic heart disease
- [ ] **c** cardiomyopathy
- [ ] **d** hypertension
- [ ] **e** atropine administration

126 There is a recognised association between ulcerative colitis and:

- [ ] **a** hepatic cirrhosis
- [ ] **b** iritis
- [ ] **c** finger clubbing
- [ ] **d** arthritis
- [ ] **e** cholangitis

127 Endocrine syndromes associated with primary bronchogenic carcinoma include:

- **a** inappropriate ADH secretion
- **b** hyperglycaemia
- **c** thyrotoxicosis
- **d** hyperparathyroidism
- **e** carcinoid syndrome

128 Pleural effusion is a common complication of:

- **a** streptococcal pneumonia
- **b** staphylococcal pneumonia
- **c** mycoplasma pneumonia
- **d** pneumococcal pneumonia
- **e** viral pneumonia

129 In primary adrenocortical failure:

- **a** blood cortisol is low
- **b** plasma ACTH is unchanged
- **c** serum potassium is low
- **d** serum sodium is low
- **e** blood glucose is low

130 You would expect to find sensory changes in the following conditions:

- **a** syringomyelia
- **b** poliomyelitis
- **c** tabes dorsalis
- **d** motor neurone disease
- **e** carpal tunnel syndrome

131 The metabolic response to major surgery includes:

- **a** an increased utilisation of glucose with a reduction in fasting blood sugar
- **b** a reduction in the amount of sodium excreted in the urine
- **c** a decrease in the circulating free fatty acids
- **d** an increased excretion of potassium in the urine
- **e** a moderate increase in oxygen consumption

132 In a patient with renal failure, if given repeatedly, the following drugs or their active metabolites are more likely to accumulate than in a normal person:

- **a** vecuronium
- **b** morphine
- **c** propofol
- **d** thiopental
- **e** erythromycin

133 Hepatitis B infection:

- **a** is transmitted by droplets
- **b** is highly contagious
- **c** is common in intravenous drug users
- **d** can be prevented by immunisation
- **e** predisposes to carcinoma of the liver

134 Radiological evidence of enlargement of the pulmonary artery is a recognised feature of:

- **a** atrial septal defect
- **b** persistent ductus arteriosus
- **c** mitral stenosis
- **d** Fallot's tetralogy
- **e** Eisenmenger's complex

135 **The following are recognised causes of thrombocytopenia:**

] **a** systemic lupus erythematosus
] **b** infectious mononucleosis
] **c** cirrhosis of the liver
] **d** treatment with a thiazide diuretic
] **e** splenectomy

136 **The carcinoid syndrome is associated with elevated plasma levels of:**

] **a** adrenaline
] **b** insulin
] **c** glucagon
] **d** prostaglandins
] **e** serotonin

137 **Clinical findings consistent with persistent vomiting for two months include:**

] **a** vitamin B_{12} deficiency anaemia
] **b** a blood urea of 12 mmol L^{-1}
] **c** hypokalaemia
] **d** hypochloraemia
] **e** tetany

138 **Ankylosing spondylitis:**

] **a** over the age of 40, occurs more commonly in women than men
] **b** is associated with low grade pyrexia
] **c** may present as sciatica
] **d** may be complicated by arthropathy affecting the hips
] **e** may be complicated by iritis

139 The following may relieve severe pain from osseous metastases of carcinoma of the prostate:

] **a** orchidectomy
] **b** short wave diathermy
] **c** stilboestrol
] **d** testosterone
] **e** radiotherapy

140 Subarachnoid haemorrhage:

] **a** causes an increase in intracranial pressure
] **b** is associated with a maximal incidence of vasospasm from the third to the tenth day after the bleed
] **c** can be detected on a CT scan
] **d** is more common in males
] **e** is precipitated by dehydration

141 Patients with acromegaly have a:

] **a** sensitivity to insulin
] **b** normal life expectancy
] **c** greater incidence of laryngeal stenosis
] **d** basophil adenoma
] **e** greater incidence of colonic cancer

142 The following are true of osmosis:

] **a** osmolarity refers to the number of osmoles per litre of water
] **b** osmolality refers to the number of osmoles per litre of specific solvent
] **c** the depression of freezing point of a solution is inversely proportional to its osmolality
] **d** Raoult's law states that the depression or lowering of vapour pressure of a solvent is proportional to the molar concentration of the solute
] **e** osmometers can also work on the principle of vapour pressure depression

143 In a time-cycled ventilator providing constant pressure generation during the inspiratory phase:

- [ ] **a** a source driving gas at 4 bar is required
- [ ] **b** the tidal volume is largely unaffected by leaks around the tracheal tube
- [ ] **c** an exponential inspiratory flow waveform is produced
- [ ] **d** the tidal volume is unaffected by changes in lung compliance
- [ ] **e** the peak inspiratory pressure is an indication of airways resistance

144 Applications of the Doppler effect in clinical practice involve measurement of a change in:

- [ ] **a** electrical conductivity of a moving stream of blood
- [ ] **b** frequency response of the arterial wall
- [ ] **c** frequency of reflected ultrasonic waves
- [ ] **d** temperature of blood as it moves peripherally
- [ ] **e** harmonic waves of reflected arterial pulses

145 Gas properties that influence resistance during laminar flow include:

- [ ] **a** critical temperature
- [ ] **b** viscosity
- [ ] **c** density
- [ ] **d** diffusion rate
- [ ] **e** molecular weight

146 FEV_1/FVC ratio measurement is useful in the detection of:

- [ ] **a** restrictive pulmonary lesions
- [ ] **b** increased functional residual capacity
- [ ] **c** obstructive pulmonary disease
- [ ] **d** inspiratory flow rate
- [ ] **e** changes in the elastic recoil of the lung

147 Potential complications of radial artery cannulation for continuous measurement of arterial blood pressure include:

- **a** fatal haemorrhage
- **b** cerebral arterial emboli
- **c** distal limb necrosis
- **d** pulmonary oedema
- **e** anaesthesia of the thenar eminence

148 In cardiac output measurement by thermodilution:

- **a** the thermistor is accurate to 0.1°C
- **b** measurements under read after 48 hours in place
- **c** the thermistor measures true 'core' temperature
- **d** measurements under read during inspiration
- **e** the thermistor bead is proximal to the balloon

149 Carbon dioxide crosses biological membranes 20 times more readily than oxygen because carbon dioxide:

- **a** has a higher Reynolds number than oxygen
- **b** is more soluble than oxygen in body fluids
- **c** has a greater molecular weight than oxygen
- **d** has a different electric charge from oxygen
- **e** is actively transported across biological membranes

150 Calculation of systemic vascular resistance requires measurement of:

- **a** coronary blood flow
- **b** pulmonary artery pressure
- **c** mean arterial blood pressure
- **d** cardiac output
- **e** rate of peripheral arteriolar flow

151 Helium:

- **a** has a viscosity similar to oxygen
- **b** is stored as a liquid in cylinders
- **c** increases vocal pitch when breathed
- **d** decreases the work of breathing in bronchospasm
- **e** supports combustion

152 Vacuum insulated evaporators (VIE) containing liquid oxygen:

- **a** store oxygen below its critical temperature of around -183°C
- **b** create a pressure of 1055 kPa if no oxygen is used
- **c** display the amount of the oxygen present as a weight
- **d** warm the oxygen when a little oxygen is drawn off
- **e** convert one volume of liquid at 15°C and atmospheric pressure to over 800 times the volume as gas

153 The pneumotachograph:

- **a** directly measures pressure change across a resistance
- **b** must have a resistance of sufficient diameter to ensure laminar gas flow
- **c** is suitable for accurate breath-by-breath monitoring
- **d** accuracy is affected by temperature change
- **e** accuracy is unaffected by alterations in gas composition

154 Intra-operative heat loss due to convection may be minimised by:

- **a** increasing the ambient theatre temperature
- **b** increasing theatre humidity
- **c** humidifying inspired gas
- **d** the use of a heated mattress
- **e** the avoidance of evaporation of spirit-based skin preparations

155 When the statistical P value is reported as being < 0.001:

-] **a** there is less than one chance in 1,000 that differences between two sample means could have occurred by chance
-] **b** the distribution of the measured variable is normal
-] **c** the null hypothesis is rejected
-] **d** the difference between two sample means is not statistically significant
-] **e** the results are clinically significant

156 In a circle breathing system:

-] **a** the capacity of the soda lime container should equal the patient's ideal tidal volume
-] **b** adequate function can be obtained with one uni-directional valve
-] **c** the adjustable pressure relief valve is best situated between the patient and the soda lime container
-] **d** the size of the reservoir bag is not critical
-] **e** any vaporiser included in the circuit should be placed between the fresh gas inlet and the patient

157 Measurement of peak expiratory flow rate:

-] **a** reveals a normal diurnal variation of less than 10%
-] **b** is usually made using a Vitalograph
-] **c** with a Wright peak flow meter uses the principle of a constant orifice with a variable pressure drop
-] **d** can be achieved using a 'rapid' capnograph
-] **e** produces a reading which is normal at 450–650 L min^{-1} in the adult

158 Oxygen concentrators:

-] **a** contain aluminium silicate
-] **b** produce at least 92% oxygen
-] **c** cannot be used in aircraft
-] **d** can be used to supply a hospital with oxygen
-] **e** provide a gas with a concentration of argon lower than air

159 The air in an operating theatre:

- a has a dew point of 37°C
- b is tested for pollution with anaesthetic gases by means of infra-red analysis
- c should be used in the calibration of an oxygen analyser
- d has a higher PO_2 when the temperature is raised
- e should undergo a statutory minimum of 15 changes per hour

160 The end-tidal partial pressure of carbon dioxide:

- a may be overestimated if measured by infra-red absorption in the presence of nitrous oxide
- b may be overestimated if measured by mass spectrometry in the presence of nitrous oxide
- c may be underestimated if measured by mass spectrometry in the presence of water vapour
- d during IPPV will be a more accurate estimate of arterial PCO_2 if positive end-expiratory pressure is applied
- e exceeds the arterial PCO_2 if the patient is in the prone position

161 On the day of major abdominal surgery, a normal adult will have:

- a his calorie requirement supplied by 1.5 litres of 5% dextrose in water
- b his daily potassium requirement supplied by 2 litres of Hartmann's solution
- c a maximum urinary osmolarity of 700 mosmol L^{-1}
- d 800 mOsm of solute which the kidneys must excrete
- e a maintenance fluid requirement of 10 ml kg^{-1} h^{-1}

162 Likely findings in an elderly dehydrated patient with prolonged intestinal obstruction who is hypotensive, tachypnoeic and confused, breathing air include:

- a hypomagnesaemia
- b low arterial oxygen saturation
- c metabolic acidosis
- d uraemia
- e hyperglycaemia

163 **Pre-operative preparation of a patient with primary hyperparathyroidism will necessitate the use of:**

- **a** 0.9% sodium chloride
- **b** furosemide
- **c** 10% dextrose
- **d** vitamin D
- **e** hydrocortisone

164 **Airway characteristics of an adult with acromegaly include:**

- **a** increased patency of the oropharynx and nasopharynx
- **b** small aperture between the vocal cords
- **c** under-development of the oral and nasopharyngeal structures
- **d** increased distance from the upper incisors to the larynx
- **e** subglottic stenosis

165 **The success of cricoid pressure in preventing aspiration into the lungs during a rapid sequence induction depends upon:**

- **a** a complete cricoid cartilage
- **b** absence of a nasogastric tube
- **c** an extended neck
- **d** compressing the oesophagus against a vertebral body
- **e** pre-oxygenation for five minutes before induction

166 **If the rapid intravenous administration of thiopental and succinylcholine is followed within one minute by the onset of muscle stiffness, the differential diagnosis should include:**

- **a** atypical plasma cholinesterase
- **b** myotonia congenita
- **c** familial periodic paralysis
- **d** malignant hyperthermia
- **e** motor neurone disease

167 **Features of pulmonary function after upper abdominal surgery include:**

- **a** a reduction in functional residual capacity of up to 50%
- **b** a decreased respiratory rate
- **c** the maintenance of normal values with effective pain relief
- **d** a shift of the majority of ventilation to the apices of the lungs
- **e** abnormal diaphragmatic function

168 **In induced hypothermia:**

- **a** MAC decreases by approximately 7% per °C reduction in temperature
- **b** there is a significant risk of ventricular fibrillation at 32°C
- **c** the oxyhaemoglobin dissociation curve is shifted to the right
- **d** the pulmonary vasoconstrictor response to hypoxia is decreased
- **e** urine output falls

169 **To repair lacerations on the palm of the hand the following nerves must be blocked:**

- **a** musculo-cutaneous
- **b** ulnar
- **c** medial cutaneous nerve of forearm
- **d** median
- **e** radial

170 **Compartment syndrome:**

- **a** occurs only in the lower limb
- **b** is not painful when muscles are passively stretched
- **c** is manifest by paraesthesia in a peripheral nerve distribution
- **d** is not compatible with the presence of a palpable distal pulse
- **e** cannot be diagnosed by observing capillary refill

171 Fat embolism syndrome:

- ❏ **a** arterial hypoxaemia is an early presenting feature
- ❏ **b** most frequently presents with respiratory symptoms and signs
- ❏ **c** causes a petechial rash usually on the conjunctiva, oral mucous membranes and skin folds of the neck and axillae
- ❏ **d** is frequently associated with focal neurological signs such as hemiparesis
- ❏ **e** is most common following lower limb fractures

172 Nitric oxide:

- ❏ **a** has a high affinity for haemoglobin
- ❏ **b** is synthesised in the body from aspartate
- ❏ **c** is a bronchodilator
- ❏ **d** shows significant tachyphylaxis
- ❏ **e** is used therapeutically at 10–100 ppm

173 Toxic effects of oxygen therapy include:

- ❏ **a** corneal ulceration
- ❏ **b** convulsions
- ❏ **c** reduced pulmonary diffusing capacity
- ❏ **d** bronchospasm
- ❏ **e** bone marrow depression

174 Intra-abdominal pressure in excess of 25 mmHg (abdominal compartment syndrome):

- ❏ **a** causes lymphoedema in the lower limbs
- ❏ **b** if untreated will cause renal failure
- ❏ **c** is effectively treated by a nasogastric tube on free drainage
- ❏ **d** requires aggressive fluid resuscitation
- ❏ **e** has a reduced mortality if surgical decompression is performed

175 **The radial nerve:**

- **a** lies lateral to the radial artery at the wrist
- **b** innervates the deltoid muscle
- **c** innervates the triceps muscle
- **d** has no sensory branches
- **e** produces dorsiflexion of the wrist joint

176 **In the fetal circulation:**

- **a** the umbilical arteries originate from the internal iliac arteries
- **b** the umbilical arteries convey de-oxygenated blood to the placenta
- **c** there are two umbilical veins
- **d** all the blood returning to the fetus passes through the fetal liver
- **e** ductus arteriosus closure is normally complete by 24 hours after delivery

177 **Pain in the area of an upper arm tourniquet is mediated via the:**

- **a** circumflex nerve
- **b** musculo-cutaneous nerve
- **c** suprascapular nerve
- **d** intercostobrachial nerve
- **e** ulnar nerve

178 **Angiotensin converting enzyme inhibitors cause:**

- **a** peripheral vasodilation
- **b** cough
- **c** increased total body water
- **d** a decreased pressor response to tracheal intubation
- **e** angioedema

179 Hepatic blood flow decreases:

- **a** during anaesthesia with isoflurane
- **b** in proportion to a decrease in hepatic oxygen consumption
- **c** during spinal anaesthesia
- **d** during propofol infusion
- **e** when the patient is placed in the lateral position

180 The following are true of the use of dibucaine in the detection of abnormal serum cholinesterase:

- **a** dibucaine inhibits serum cholinesterase
- **b** 97% of the population possess the normal enzyme
- **c** in patients homozygous for the atypical enzyme, the dibucaine number is in excess of 80
- **d** in the 3% of patients who are heterozygous for the abnormal enzyme, the dibucaine number is approximately 55
- **e** fluoride is used as an alternative enzyme inhibitor

MCQ examination Single Best Answer (SBA)

SBA Paper 1

Question 1

A neonate born at 28 weeks gestation and now six weeks old develops apnoeic episodes following an inguinal herniotomy performed under GA.

Which of the following blood results/vital signs are *LEAST* likely to be associated with apnoeic spells in this age group?

a blood glucose 1.7 mmol L^{-1}

b core temperature 35.2°C

c core temperature 39.5°C

d haemoglobin 11.5 g dl^{-1}

e serum ionised calcium 0.8 mmol L^{-1}

Question 2

A 37-year-old man has an uneventful total colectomy performed under GA. Surgery, lasting five hours, was performed in the Lloyd Davis position. One hour post-operatively, with a 0.1% L-bupivacaine thoracic epidural infusion in progress, he has no abdominal pain but does have pain in both calves. There are decreased lower limb movements bilaterally with reduced pinprick sensation in all dermatomes below the knees.

What is the most appropriate initial investigation in this scenario?

a compartment pressure measurement in both calves

b doppler arterial pulse measurement in both legs

c electromyography of leg flexor and extensor muscles

d magnetic resonance imaging of the thoraco-lumbar spine

e ultrasound scan of deep venous system in both calves

Question 3

A previously fit 54-year-old woman presents to the Emergency Department with severe sore throat and increasingly noisy breathing for the past 12 hours. She finds it difficult to swallow her saliva and cannot tolerate lying flat. Her tympanic temperature is 39.2°C, pulse rate 110 beats min^{-1}, BP 130/85, SpO_2 92% on 35% oxygen via facemask. There is marked inspiratory stridor.

What is the most appropriate management plan?

a administer intravenous steroids and antibiotics, nebulised adrenaline and high flow oxygen by CPAP facemask in a high dependency area

b after direct examination of the oropharynx, the patient should have blood cultures taken, receive oral antibiotics, high flow oxygen and be observed in a high dependency area

c the airway should be secured by awake fibreoptic intubation under local anaesthesia, followed by admission to an Intensive Care Unit

d the airway should be secured by tracheal intubation following direct laryngoscopy under deep inhalational anaesthesia

e the patient should be transferred, fully monitored, to the operating theatre for immediate tracheostomy under local anaesthesia

Question 4

A 7-year-old child weighing 24 kg is having squint correction surgery under general anaesthesia. During the procedure, his heart rate falls abruptly to 45 beats per minute and his blood pressure is 70/40.

What is the most appropriate initial action to take?

a ask the surgeon to release the globe of the eye

b give atropine 480 μg intravenously

c give ephedrine 6 mg intravenously

d give glycopyrollate 240 μg intravenously

e reduce the inspired concentration of sevoflurane

Question 5

A 45-year-old woman with a past history of mild asthma and anxiety undergoes left shoulder arthroscopic surgery under interscalene brachial plexus block. Post-operatively she complains of dyspnoea and light-headedness. Breath sounds are slightly reduced on the left side of the chest. SpO_2 92% (on air), BP 110/70, peak flow 290 L min^{-1}. A standard portable CXR appears normal.

What is the most likely cause of her symptoms?

a exacerbation of asthma

b left phrenic nerve palsy

c left recurrent laryngeal nerve palsy

d psychogenic dyspnoea

e subarachnoid local anaesthetic injection

Question 6

A 72-year-old man is ventilated on ICU four hours following elective coronary artery surgery. His pulse is 110 beats min^{-1}, BP 85/45, CVP 17 mmHg, urine output 25 ml hr^{-1} in the last two hours and tympanic temperature 37.6°C. Heart sounds are difficult to hear but breath sounds are normal. A 12-lead ECG is unchanged from pre-operatively.

What is the most likely cause of the patient's current clinical condition?

a developing septic shock

b hypovolaemia

c myocardial ischaemia

d pericardial tamponade

e tension pneumothorax

Question 7

A 56-year-old woman who had a total colectomy develops a tachyarrhythmia 12 hours post-operatively on the HDU. She has a past history of hypertension treated by bendroflumethiazide but no history of cardiac problems.

Which of the following serum electrolyte abnormalities is the most likely to contribute to the arrhythmia?

a ionised calcium 1.88 mmol L^{-1}

b magnesium 0.38 mmol L^{-1}

c phosphate 0.58 mmol L^{-1}

d potassium 3.4 mmol L^{-1}

e sodium 129 mmol L^{-1}

Question 8

You need to anaesthetise a woman who does not speak English, for a category 3 Caesarean section.

What is the best way to take a history and provide information to this patient?

a professional telephone translation service

b the O and G registrar who has some understanding of the patient's language

c the patient's husband who has a limited command of English

d the patient's 11-year-old daughter who is bilingual

e written translated materials

Question 9

A 10-month-old apparently well infant presents for religious circumcision under GA. Routine examination reveals a soft systolic murmur; the rest of the examination is normal.

The most appropriate action to take is:

a postpone surgery and obtain an urgent cardiac echo

b postpone surgery and refer the child back to the GP

c proceed with anaesthesia because this is an 'innocent' murmur

d proceed with anaesthesia giving antibiotic cover

e proceed with surgery under local anaesthesia

Question 10

You administer a general anaesthetic to a previously fit young man for arthroscopic repair of a ruptured left anterior cruciate ligament. The thigh tourniquet was inflated to 200 mmHg above the systolic blood pressure for 110 minutes. Post-operatively, he complains of paraesthesiae in his left calf and sole of the foot.

Which of the following is the single most likely cause of the paraesthesiae?

a compartment syndrome in the thigh

b compression injury to the sciatic nerve

c deep venous thrombosis in the calf

d ischaemic injury to the calf muscles

e pressure injury from the edge of the operating table

Question 11

A 40-year-old man is scheduled for elective knee arthroscopy. You commence intravenous induction with thiopental but after injecting 100 mg the patient complains of an intense burning pain in his hand associated with blanching of the fingers.

What is the most important next step to take in managing this situation?

a arrange for a stellate ganglion block to be performed in the affected limb

b insert an IV cannula in the contralateral limb and administer opioid analgesia

c insert an IV cannula in the contralateral limb and administer papaverine

d leave the IV cannula *in situ* and flush with heparinised saline

e remove the IV cannula, apply local pressure and elevate the limb

Question 12

A 75-year-old man is scheduled for a total knee replacement under general anaesthesia supplemented by a femoral nerve block for peri-operative analgesia.

What is the most effective way to reduce the likelihood of local anaesthetic toxicity during placement of the block?

a adding a vasoconstrictor to the local anaesthetic

b injecting the local anaesthetic slowly and aspirating at regular intervals

c monitoring the patient with ECG, SpO_2 and non-invasive blood pressure

d not exceeding the maximum permissible dose of local anaesthetic

e using a nerve stimulator to guide block placement

Question 13

A 60-year-old man is scheduled for a palmar fasciectomy. He has angina, with several episodes of chest pain each week and says that he is 'allergic to local anaesthetics'. Fifteen years ago he had a local anaesthetic block at the dentist, following which he developed palpitations and became very anxious for 10–15 minutes.

Which is the most likely explanation for his previous experience at the dentist?

a adverse reaction to adrenaline absorbed from the local anaesthetic solution

b anaphylactic reaction to a preservative in the local anaesthetic solution

c episode of angina brought on by the stress of the situation

d systemic toxicity due to accidental intravascular injection of local anaesthetic

e systemic toxicity due to overdose of local anaesthetic

Question 14

An otherwise fit 80-year-old man had uneventful resection of a bladder tumour under general anaesthesia. A three-way irrigating urinary catheter is inserted at the end of the procedure. In recovery, he looks pale and has severe abdominal discomfort. His pulse rate is 48 beats min^{-1} and blood pressure is 75/30. The drained irrigating fluid appears clear.

What is the most appropriate action that would resolve the clinical situation in this patient?

a atropine 0.3 mg IV bolus

b ephedrine 6 mg IV bolus

c flush the 3-way catheter

d morphine 5 mg IV bolus

e rapid infusion of 500 ml 0.9% saline

Question 15

A patient develops anaphylactic shock shortly after induction of general anaesthesia, is treated with intravenous adrenaline and makes an uneventful recovery.

Which is the best explanation of the therapeutic action of adrenaline in the treatment of anaphylaxis?

a causes increased myocardial contractility and bronchodilation

b causes increased myocardial contractility and tachycardia

c causes peripheral vasoconstriction and decreases mast cell degranulation

d causes peripheral vasoconstriction and increased myocardial contractility

e causes tachycardia and decreases mast cell degranulation

Question 16

A previously fit 60-year-old woman is oliguric (< 0.5 ml kg^{-1} hr^{-1}) 48 hours after a laparotomy for colonic carcinoma. Laboratory testing of her urine reveals the following:

Specific gravity = 1.020
Sodium 2 mmol L^{-1}
Osmolarity 600 mosmol L^{-1}

What is the most likely diagnosis?

a acute tubular necrosis

b analgesic nephropathy

c hypovolaemia

d renal calculi

e bilateral ureteric injury

Question 17

A 59-year-old man with a caecal carcinoma requiring a right hemicolectomy has been referred for pre-operative assessment. Following an episode of crescendo angina three months previously he had a coronary angioplasty and multiple coronary stent insertion. He is currently well with no further angina and he is taking aspirin and clopidogrel.

What would be the most appropriate management plan for this patient?

a continue both anti-platelet drugs and give a pre-operative platelet transfusion

b postpone surgery until he has completed his anti-platelet therapy

c schedule urgent surgery and continue both anti-platelet drugs peri-operatively

d stop aspirin for seven days pre-operatively but continue clopidogrel

e stop clopidogrel for seven days pre-operatively but continue aspirin

Question 18

A 64-year-old man with a BMI of 41 kg m^{-2} had a laparotomy for resection of hepatic metastases one hour ago. In the recovery room his SpO_2 is 85% breathing room air, but 98% when supplemental oxygen is delivered by nasal prongs at 2 L min^{-1}.

Which is the most likely explanation for his current respiratory status?

a alveolar atelectasis

b alveolar hypoventilation

c diffusion hypoxia due to nitrous oxide use

d residual neuromuscular blockade

e residual inhalational anaesthesia

Question 19

Lumbar chemical sympathectomy has a variety of potential therapeutic indications.

Which condition has the best chance of sustained improvement with this technique?

- **a** complex regional pain syndrome type I
- **b** hyperhydrosis
- **c** intermittent claudication
- **d** ischaemic rest pain in the foot
- **e** venous ulceration around the ankle

Question 20

An 18-year-old male patient is admitted to a district hospital with an isolated severe head injury and is promptly intubated, ventilated and sedated. Soon afterwards his SpO_2 is 99% (FiO_2 0.5), $ETCO_2$ 4.5 kPa, BP 200/120, pulse 44 beats min^{-1} and he has a fixed dilated left pupil.

What is the most appropriate next action to take?

- **a** actively cool the patient to 35°C
- **b** arrange an urgent head CT scan
- **c** arrange transfer to the nearest neurosurgical unit
- **d** insert an arterial line
- **e** prescribe an intravenous bolus of mannitol 0.5 g kg^{-1}

Question 21

You are called to the Emergency Department to see a previously well 20-year-old woman who has been admitted following a grand mal fit outside a nightclub. After administration of lorazepam she stops fitting and is now not responsive to commands. Her SpO_2 is 94% on air and blood glucose is 4.5 mmol L^{-1}. No other history is available.

What is the next most useful investigation you would perform on this patient?

- **a** arterial blood gases
- **b** blood alcohol level
- **c** drug toxicology screen
- **d** full blood count
- **e** serum electrolytes

Question 22

A 78-year-old woman has had severe, lancinating episodes of pain below the right eye for four months which are sometimes triggered by face washing. Carbamazepine in full doses has produced little improvement in her pain. She has a past history of hypertension and transient ischaemic episodes.

What therapeutic intervention should be considered next?

a gabapentin

b microvascular decompression surgery

c slow-release oral morphine

d rhizolysis of the trigeminal ganglion

e amitryptyline

Question 23

A previously fit 70-year-old man undergoes radical neck dissection for malignant disease. The patient is stable until the surgeon dissects the tumour away from the carotid sheath. Suddenly, the systolic BP falls from 110 mmHg to 60 mmHg, heart rate increases to 110 beats min^{-1}, SpO_2 falls to 87% and end tidal CO_2 concentration falls to 1.9 kPa.

What is the most likely cause for the change in vital signs?

a anaphylactic shock

b carotid sinus manipulation

c myocardial ischaemia

d tension pneumothorax

e venous air embolism

Question 24

A previously fit 5-year-old child is distressed and in severe pain in the recovery room following emergency appendicectomy. He is awake and cardiovascularly stable. Intra-operatively, he received fentanyl 3 µg kg^{-1} IV, paracetamol 15 mg kg^{-1} IV and diclofenac 1 mg kg^{-1} PR.

What would be the most appropriate management option now?

a administer Entonox until the child's mother arrives

b codeine phosphate 1 mg kg^{-1} intramuscularly

c codeine phosphate 1 mg kg^{-1} orally

d commence a Nurse-Controlled Analgesia (NCA) pump using morphine

e morphine 0.1 mg kg^{-1} IV bolus

Question 25

A 26-year-old primigravida (BMI = 47) with a twin pregnancy is in established labour at 38 weeks gestation. She requests an epidural for pain relief but on inserting the epidural needle at L 3, 4 an accidental dural puncture occurs.

What is the most appropriate action to take?

a abandon the epidural and use inhalational analgesia

b abandon the epidural and use opioid-based analgesia

c insert the epidural catheter intrathecally and use it for spinal analgesia

d perform an epidural blood patch to prevent post-dural puncture headache

e resite the epidural at an adjacent spinal interspace

Question 26

A 70-year-old woman had a gastrectomy 48 hours ago and she has a thoracic epidural for post-operative analgesia which is functioning well. Warfarin, for atrial fibrillation, was stopped seven days ago and she was converted to low molecular weight heparin. Clotting studies and platelet count are in the normal range. Today she is noted to have a white, cold left leg.

What is the most appropriate initial management?

a doppler studies of the arterial supply of the left leg

b increase the dose of low molecular weight heparin

c organise an urgent MRI scan of the spine

d top up the epidural with her lying on the left side

e ultrasound of the deep veins of the lower limbs

Question 27

A 64-year-old man presents to the Emergency Department with an exacerbation of COPD.

His arterial blood gases breathing air show the following:

pH 7.30
pO_2 5.5 kPa
pCO_2 7.5 kPa
HCO_3 35 mmol L^{-1}
Hb 18.5 g dl^{-1}

Which is the most appropriate device to initiate oxygen therapy?

a Hudson mask

b MC mask

c nasal prongs

d non-rebreathing reservoir mask

e Venturi mask

Question 28

A 35-year-old male suffered a severe isolated traumatic brain injury ten days ago. There is no neurological recovery or respiratory effort 48 hours after cessation of propofol sedation and neuromuscular blockade with atracurium. The serum sodium concentration is 152 mmol L^{-1}, core temperature is 37.5°C; serum glucose concentration is normal. The patient's family know that brain stem death is suspected.

What is the most appropriate action to take now?

a consult the organ donor register

b cool the patient to 36.5°C

c perform an EEG

d reduce serum sodium below 150 mmol L^{-1}

e undertake brain stem death tests

Question 29

A 70-year-old patient with a long history of severe depression and hypertension is admitted as an emergency with severe peritonitis. He is taking bendroflumethiazide, enalapril and phenelzine. During laparotomy, his blood pressure falls to 65/30 mmHg and heart rate rises to 100 beats min^{-1}. There is no cardiovascular improvement in response to a fluid bolus which raises the CVP to +10 mmHg.

Which is the most appropriate initial pharmacological intervention?

a ephedrine

b metaraminol

c noradrenaline

d phenylephrine

e vasopressin

Question 30

A 19-year-old man is listed for a cervical lymph node biopsy after a six-week history of generalised lymphadenopathy and intermittent pyrexia. He is breathless on mild exertion and needs to sleep with four pillows.

Which is the most important pre-operative investigation that will influence your anaesthetic management?

a CT scan of the neck

b CXR

c full blood count

d flow volume loops

e spirometry

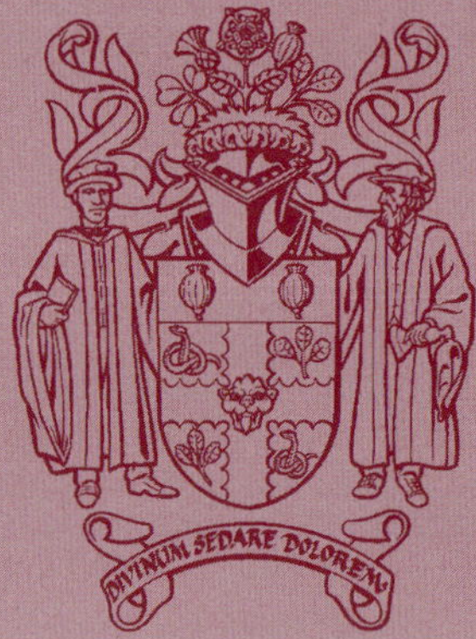
DIVINUM SEDARE DOLOREM

SOE examination

Clinical Anaesthesia – Long Cases

Case 1

Information given to candidate

A 60-year-old lady who is taking non-steroidal anti-inflammatory drugs for osteoarthritis of the hip has been in the medical ward for three days with a refractory gastrointestinal haemorrhage. She has received a total of five units of blood. In the past 24 hours her urine output has been 1,200 ml with a specific gravity of 1.030. Following a sudden further haemorrhage at 10.00 am this morning she is scheduled for emergency laparotomy.

On examination

A pale lady, lying quietly in bed.

Height 162 cm (5 ft 3 in)
Weight 65 kg
Temp 37°C
Pulse 125 bpm
BP 90/60 mmHg
Respiratory rate 20 breaths per minute

Chest dull to percussion over the left base with absent breath sounds in that region.

Throughout the rest of the chest the breath sounds are vesicular.

Apex beat palpable in 5th left interspace in the mid-clavicular line. Heart sounds normal.

Systematic examination is otherwise grossly normal.

Provided for the candidate are

1 Biochemistry results taken at 9.00 am.
2 Haematology results taken at 9.00 am.
3 Results of a coagulation screen at the same time.
4 CXR.

Clinical details GI bleeding last three days severe haematemesis this morning – for emergency surgery			*Current therapy* NSAIDs for arthritis	
Patient No	*Age*	*Sex*	*Weight*	*Date*
1	60	female	65 kg	

			Reference values	
Sodium	148	mmol L^{-1}	135–145	mmol L^{-1}
Potassium	5.0	mmol L^{-1}	3.5–5.0	mmol L^{-1}
Bicarbonate	30	mmol L^{-1}	24–31	mmol L^{-1}
Chloride	105	mmol L^{-1}	95–105	mmol L^{-1}
Urea	10.5	mmol L^{-1}	3.0–6.5	mmol L^{-1}
Creatinine	150	μmol L^{-1}	60–125	μmol L^{-1}
Calcium		mmol L^{-1}	2.15–2.55	mmol L^{-1}
Phosphate		mmol L^{-1}	0.7–1.5	mmol L^{-1}
Total Protein		g L^{-1}	63–80	g L^{-1}
Albumin		g L^{-1}	32–50	g L^{-1}
T Bilirubin		μmol L^{-1}	< 17	μmol L^{-1}
ALP (Alk Phos)		IU L^{-1}	100–300	IU L^{-1}
AST		IU L^{-1}	5–42	IU L^{-1}
Glucose (random)		mmol L^{-1}	2.5–6.0 (fasting)	mmol L^{-1}

Clinical details GI bleeding for three days severe haematemesis this morning – for emergency surgery			*Current therapy* NSAIDs for arthritis	
Patient No	*Age*	*Sex*	*Weight*	*Date*
1	60	female	65 kg	

		Reference values
Hb	11 g dl^{-1}	15 ± 2 g dL^{-1}
RBC	4.4 x 10^{12} L^{-1}	5.0 ± 0.8 x 10^{12} L^{-1}
PCV	0.38	0.45 ± 0.05
MCH	27.5 pg	29 ± 2 pg
MCHC	32%	34 ± 2%
MCV	86 fl	87 ± 5 fl
Platelets	80 x 10^9 L^{-1}	150–400 x 10^9 L^{-1}
WBC	8.2 x 10^9 L^{-1}	7.0 ± 3 x 10^9 L^{-1}
gran	**72%**	
lymph	**18%**	
mono	**9%**	
eosin	**–**	

Clinical details GI bleeding for three days severe haematemesis this morning – for emergency surgery			*Current therapy* NSAIDs for arthritis	
Patient No	*Age*	*Sex*	*Weight*	*Date*
1	60	female	65 kg	
			Reference values	
Coagulation screen Prothrombin time (PT)				
	patient =	16 sec		
	control =	12 sec		
INR	=	1.7	1–1.3	
KCCT	=	63 sec	35–45 (control)	
Fibrinogen	=	$0.9\ g\ L^{-1}$	1.5–4.0 (control)	

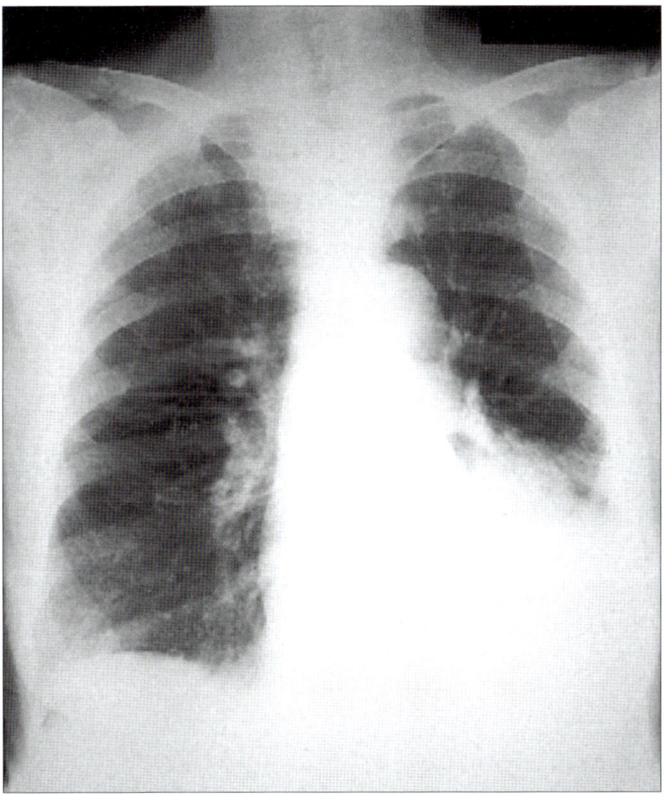

Case 2

Information given to candidate

A 7-year-old boy has been admitted with a history of a painful swelling in the right side of his scrotum which was first noticed six hours ago. He has been diagnosed as having torsion of the right testis. His last oral intake was five hours ago and he has vomited several times. He has had a chronic cough for the last ten days.

Past medical history

He has suffered from asthma for three years for which he uses inhaled beclomethasone 100 μg twice daily and a salbutamol inhaler (dose 200 μg) during attacks. He has been admitted to hospital several times with acute attacks of asthma following chest infections.

On examination

A quiet frightened child, lying still in bed; he is pale and sweaty and in obvious pain especially when coughing.

Height 105 cm (3 ft 3 in)
Weight 30 kg
Temp 38.5°C
Pulse rate 112 bpm regular
BP 100/70 mmHg
Respiratory rate 24 breaths per minute

Left lung base is dull to percussion and with reduced air entry on auscultation. Rhonchi are audible throughout both lungs with scattered moist sounds.

Heart sounds normal.

Systematic examination is otherwise grossly normal.

Provided for the candidate are:

1 Biochemistry results

2 Haematology results

3 CXR

Clinical details 7-year-old boy asthmatic, for theatre			*Current therapy* Beclomethasone inhaler Salbutamol inhaler	
Patient No	*Age*	*Sex*	*Weight*	*Date*
2	7	male	30 kg	

			Reference values	
Sodium	138	mmol L^{-1}	135–145	mmol L^{-1}
Potassium	4.1	mmol L^{-1}	3.5–5.0	mmol L^{-1}
Bicarbonate	25	mmol L^{-1}	24–31	mmol L^{-1}
Chloride	99	mmol L^{-1}	95–105	mmol L^{-1}
Urea	3.2	mmol L^{-1}	3.0–6.5	mmol L^{-1}
Creatinine	84	µmol L^{-1}	60–125	µmol L^{-1}
Calcium		mmol L^{-1}	2.15–2.55	mmol L^{-1}
Phosphate		mmol L^{-1}	0.7–1.5	mmol L^{-1}
Total Protein		g L^{-1}	63–80	g L^{-1}
Albumin		g L^{-1}	32–50	g L^{-1}
Bilirubin		µmol L^{-1}	< 17	µmol L^{-1}
ALP (Alk Phos)		IU L^{-1}	100–300	IU L^{-1}
ALT		IU L^{-1}	5–42	IU L^{-1}
Glucose (random)		mmol L^{-1}	2.5–6.0 (fasting)	mmol L^{-1}

Clinical details 7-year-old boy asthmatic, for theatre			*Current therapy* Beclomethasone inhaler Salbutamol inhaler	
Patient No	*Age*	*Sex*	*Weight*	*Date*
2	7	male	30 kg	

		Reference values
Hb	12.8 g dl^{-1}	13.5 ± 2 g dl^{-1}
RBC	4.9 x 10^{12} L^{-1}	5.0 ± 0.8 x 10^{12} L^{-1}
PCV	0.45	0.40 ± 0.05
MCH	29 pg	27 ± 3 pg
MCHC	32%	34 ± 2%
MCV	83 fl	87 ± 7 fl
Platelets	202 x 10^9 L^{-1}	150–400 x 10^9 L^{-1}
WBC	13.5 x 10^9 L^{-1}	8.5 ± 4.5 x 10^9 L^{-1}
gran	**67%**	
lymph	**25%**	
mono	**–%**	
eosin	**–%**	

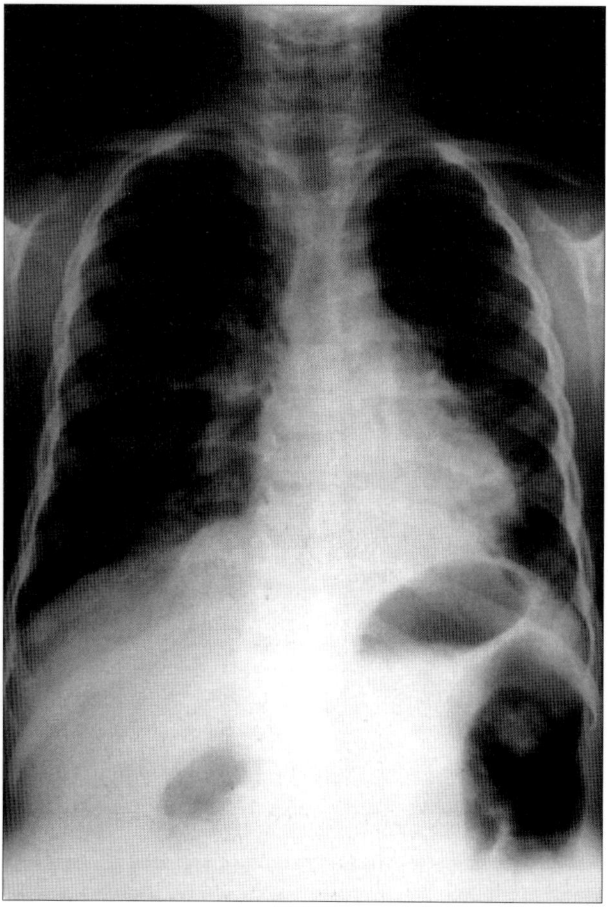

Case 3

Information given to candidate

You have been called to the Accident and Emergency Department to assess a 53-year-old woman for anaesthesia. Diagnostic peritoneal lavage has revealed blood in her abdominal cavity. She has been involved in an accident in which the car she was driving was struck by a lorry. It took some time to cut her from the wreckage. So far, no past medical history has been obtained.

On examination

The patient is conscious.

She is complaining of right-sided chest and hip pain.

She appears breathless with rapid shallow breathing and is receiving oxygen via a face mask.

An intravenous infusion is running.

She is overweight and provisionally assessed as:

Height 168 cm (5 ft 6 in)
Weight ~90 kg
Temp 36 °C
Pulse 100 bpm
BP 90/45

Respiratory rate 40 breaths per minute. Chest movements are asymmetrical with paradoxical movement of the right side.

Clinical and radiological confirmation has been obtained of fractures of the pelvis and right femur. CT scans of head and neck show no fractures or intracerebral haematoma.

Provided for the candidate are:

1 Haematology

2 Biochemistry

3 Arterial blood Gas

4 Chest X-ray

Clinical details			*Current therapy*	
RTA Fractured Pelvis and Right Femur			None	
Patient No	*Age*	*Sex*	*Weight*	*Date*
3	53	female	~ 90 kg	

			Reference values	
Sodium	141	mmol L^{-1}	135–145	mmol L^{-1}
Potassium	5.0	mmol L^{-1}	3.5–5.0	mmol L^{-1}
Bicarbonate	19	mmol L^{-1}	24–31	mmol L^{-1}
Chloride	104	mmol L^{-1}	95–105	mmol L^{-1}
Urea	7.4	mmol L^{-1}	3.0–6.5	mmol L^{-1}
Creatinine		μmol L^{-1}	60–125	μmol L^{-1}
Glucose (random)	11.4	mmol L^{-1}	2.5–6.0 (fasting)	mmol L^{-1}
Urinalysis				
Protein				
Glucose	+			
Blood				

Clinical details			*Current therapy*	
RTA Fractured Pelvis and Right Femur			None	
Patient No	*Age*	*Sex*	*Weight*	*Date*
3	53	female	~ 90 kg	

		Reference values
Hb	11.5 g dl^{-1}	15 ± 2 g dl^{-1}
RBC	4.2 x 10^{12} L^{-1}	5.0 ± 0.8 x 10^{12} L^{-1}
PCV	0.37	0.45 ± 0.05
MCH	27 pg	29 ± 2 pg
MCHC	31%	34 ± 2%
MCV	88 fl	87 ± 5 fl
Platelets	201 x 10^9 L^{-1}	150–400 x 10^9 L^{-1}
WBC	18.6 x 10^9 L^{-1}	7.0 ± 3 x 10^9 L^{-1}
gran		
lymph		
mono		
eosin		

Clinical details RTA Fractured Pelvis and Right Femur			*Current therapy* None	
Patient No	*Age*	*Sex*	*Weight*	*Date*
3	53	female	~ 90 kg	

Arterial Blood Gas Analysis			**Reference values**
pH	7.26		7.35–7.45
$PaCO_2$	4.92	kPa	4.67–6.0 kPa
PaO_2	31.8	kPa	12.0–13.3 kPa
HCO_3	16.6	mmol L^{-1}	22–26 mmol L^{-1}
Total CO	17.8	mmol L^{-1}	23–27 mmol L^{-1}
Base Excess	-8.9	mmol L^{-1}	-2 to +2
O_2 saturation	99.7%		

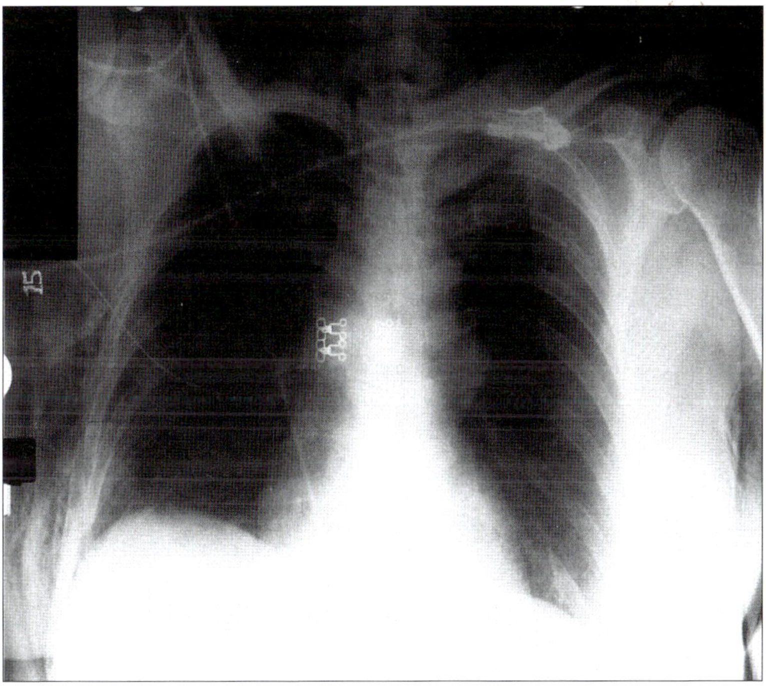

Clinical Anaesthesia – Short Cases

The cases are shown as if in a real Structured Oral Examination (SOE 1). The three questions are deliberately grouped together, as in the examination, to cover the range of the syllabus (planned and emergency anaesthetic care, core and sub-specialty practice). The individual questions cover topics of varying difficulty. Each specific question also covers a range of areas often of increasing complexity to fully explore the candidates' knowledge and understanding.

All examiners will start with the same opening question and will cover the same subject area in a question, but the SOE is an interaction between two professionals. The style, order and direction of subsequent questioning in any examination will be partly directed by the candidate's response to a previous question. The examiner will ask supplementary questions as appropriate to both clarify and explore answers given.

Candidates run through a question at different speeds. Most candidates will cover most of the areas in the allotted time. For candidates that progress through the topic quickly, due to either very good or very poor knowledge, each question has a series of topics at the end labelled 'Fillers.' These are not topics that must be covered by a candidate to pass the case, but are present to avoid those embarrassing little silences. They are included to give candidates a true reflection of the examination.

Paper 1

Question 1: Anaesthetic implications of pacemakers.
A 75-year-old man presents for gastrectomy for carcinoma. On pre-operative assessment you find he had a pacemaker fitted three years ago.
How would you proceed?

Supporting information
Nil

How would you proceed?
Possible supplementary questions:

1 He has a pacemaker card that says the pacemaker is DDD. What does this mean?
2 What are the anaesthetic implications of routine pacemakers?
3 How does the situation change if the patient has an implantable cardiac defibrillator (ICD) in place because of hypertrophic obstructive cardiomyopathy (HOCM)?

(Filler – How would you manage a failure of a standard pacemaker during the operation?)

Question 2: Septic shock in a patient admitted with cholecystitis.
The outreach nurse calls you for advice regarding a 46-year-old lady admitted to hospital two days previously with acute cholecystitis who is now hypotensive and tachycardic. What advice would you give?

Supporting information
Arterial blood gases

What advice would you give?
Possible supplementary questions:
1 What is sepsis?
2 What is the underlying pathophysiology (briefly)?
3 What would you do when you arrive on the ward?
4 What investigations would you review or request and what would you expect them to show?
5 You will be shown a set of arterial blood gases listed below and asked to interpret them.
6 Despite receiving several litres of crystalloid the patient remains hypotensive. What would you do?

(Filler: How may the cardiovascular system be monitored safely and effectively to manage this septic patient in the Intensive Care Unit?)

Arterial Blood Gas Result

		Normal Range
FIO_2	= 0.6	
pH	= 7.07	7.35–7.45
PaO_2 (kPa)	= 11.4	9.3–13.3
$PaCO_2$ (kPa)	= 1.52	4.7–6.0
HCO_3 (mmol L^{-1})	= 3.1	22–26
Base Excess	= -26.3	-3 – +3
Lactate (mmol L^{-1})	5.8	0.5–2.2

SOE **Questions**

Question 3: An Obstetric Emergency

You are resident on the Labour Suite. A 23-year-old lady who is 32 weeks pregnant is coming in by emergency ambulance. She was out shopping, went to the toilet and has part of the umbilical cord per vagina.

What would you do?

Supporting information

Nil

What would you do?

Areas to be covered in the initial and supplementary questions:

1 What would you do prior to her arrival on delivery suite?

2 She has now arrived

a What are your anaesthetic choices?

b What would you do pre-operatively?

3 Describe the anaesthetic you would undertake for this patient.

4 Discuss her post-operative care.

(Filler – The baby is born in poor condition and the paediatricians have not arrived. Describe the assessment and resuscitation of a newborn child.)

Paper 2

Question 1: Anaesthesia for surgery in a patient who is a Jehovah's Witness

You see a patient in the pre-assessment clinic who is a Jehovah's Witness. She is due to have an operative procedure with possible significant blood loss.

What specific problems does this situation pose?

Supporting information

Nil

What specific problems does this situation pose?

Possible supplementary questions:

1 How would you approach these problems in the pre-assessment clinic?

2 What principles apply per-operatively?

3 If the patient is 14 years old how would the situation change?

(Filler – How would the situation change if the patient presented unconscious requiring an emergency operation?)

Question 2: The child with stridor

You are called to the paediatric ward by your paediatric colleagues to help in the management of a 2-year-old child just admitted with stridor of recent onset. They want your advice on whether the child should be intubated.

How would you assess patency of the airway and the need for intubation?

Supporting information

Nil

How would you assess patency of the airway and the need for intubation?

Possible supplementary questions:

1 What is stridor?

2 What is your differential diagnosis?

3 Describe your initial management?

The child is toxic (temperature 38.4°C) and unimmunised. There is severe upper airway obstruction. The child is hypoxic but still breathing and you judge intubation is necessary. Describe your anaesthetic approach.

(Filler – The airway is lost on induction, and you can neither intubate nor ventilate. How do you manage this?)

Question 3: The lady with bunions

A 72-year-old lady presents for correction of bunions as a day case. On systemic enquiry she complains of aching in the right side of her chest and weight loss of one stone (7 kg) over a three month period. You arrange a pre-operative chest X-ray.

Is the CXR normal?

Supporting information

CXR 3

Is the CXR normal?

Possible supplementary questions:

1 What is the differential diagnosis?

2 She desperately wants her bunions doing, would you proceed? What would you tell her?

3 She is fully investigated and subsequently listed for an operation involving a thoracotomy (5th rib space). What are the choices for post-operative pain relief after thoracotomy?

4 How would you manage her airway for such an operation?

(Filler – What are the indications for single lung ventilation?)

Clinical Science

Anatomy

What problems may be found at pre-operative assessment in patients presenting for surgery for a pituitary tumour?

- Relevant anatomy of the pituitary
- What disorders of serum sodium may be encountered after pituitary surgery?

Physiology

What problems might result from aortic cross-clamping and how can they be reduced?

- What is meant by reperfusion injury and what is the mechanism?
- Anaesthetic best practice in open aortic surgery

Pharmacology

During a lumbar plexus block your patient complains of feeling unwell. What features would alert you to local anaesthetic toxicity?

- What are the factors which determine whether LA toxicity develops?
- What is the mechanism of action of LA toxicity?
- Management of systemic bupivacaine toxicity

Clinical measurement

What are the sources of pollution in the operating theatre?

- Concerns about anaesthetic gas pollution
- How may pollution be reduced or prevented?
- Features of a scavenging system
- Other reasons for efficient ventilation

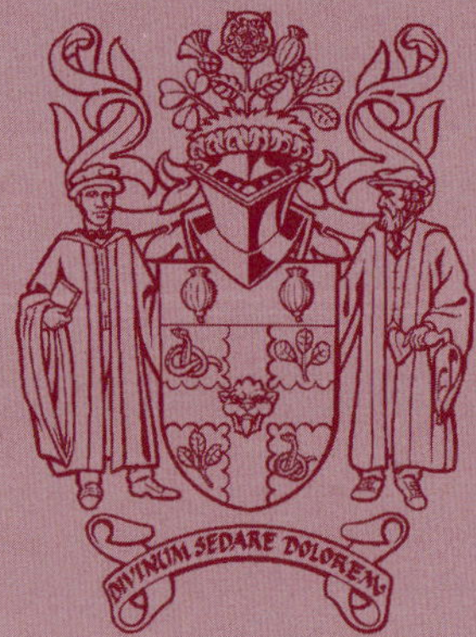
DIVINUM SEDARE DOLOREM

Section 3: Answers

DIVINUM SEDARE DOLOREM

SAQ examination

SAQ Paper 1

Question 1

a List the advantages of day case surgical management compared with inpatient care (30%)

b What are the surgical prerequisites that make a procedure suitable for day case management? (30%)

c Summarise the discharge criteria that a patient needs to meet following a day case procedure (40%)

Curriculum references: In 9.1.2 , In 9.1.6, In 16.1.2, 16.2.1 and In 18.1.3	
Answers	Marks for each (max)
a Advantages ❍ Decreased hospital acquired infection rates ❍ Decreased thrombo-embolism due to early mobilisation ❍ Less cancellations on day of surgery ❍ Less anxiety if overnight stay avoided – especially children ❍ Cost effective; operations cheaper to perform as day cases ❍ Higher throughput of patients ❍ Frees up inpatient beds for more complex cases	**6**
b Surgical prerequisites ❍ Short duration (< 2 hours) ❍ Low risk of major peri-operative haemorrhage ❍ Post-operative pain manageable with oral analgesia ❍ No ongoing requirements for post-operative IV fluids ❍ Low potential for delayed airway compromise ❍ Allows rapid mobilisation that facilitates prompt discharge ❍ No requirement for specialised post-op observations (e.g. neurological observations)	**6**
c Discharge criteria ❍ Stable vital signs ❍ Fully awake and orientated appropriate to age ❍ Pain well controlled ❍ PONV well controlled/able to tolerate oral fluids ❍ Passed urine (post urological surgery and neuraxial blocks) ❍ Able to stand, dress and ambulate (crutches/wheelchair OK) ❍ Responsible adult escort for journey home available ❍ Journey time less than two hours. ❍ Patient's home situation compatible with post-operative care (e.g. responsible adult supervision is available)	**8**

SAQ **Answers**

Question 2

a Describe the type and course of primary pain afferents from the cornea to the brain (20%).

b List the techniques which can provide local anaesthesia of the cornea (20%)

c Which muscles and their innervation need to be blocked to achieve complete akinesia of the globe? (15%)

d What are the complications (30%) of sharp needle orbital blocks and how can they be minimised? (15%)

Curriculum references: 17.1.9 – 17.1.12	
Answers	Marks for each (max)
a Course of afferents Naked nerve endings of Aδ and C fibres. Branches of the lachrymal, frontal and nasociliary nerves unite to form the ophthalmic division of the trigeminal nerve. Cell bodies lie in the semilunar ganglion and neurones pass in the fifth cranial nerve to the Pons and then terminate in the nucleus of the spinal tract.	**4**
b Techniques ○ Topical ○ Subconjuctival LA infiltration ○ Extraconal block (peribulbar) ○ Intraconal block (retrobulbar) ○ Sub-Tenon's block	**4**
c Nerves and muscles Cranial nerves III (supplies inferior, superior and medial rectus muscles), IV (supplies superior oblique muscle) and VI (supplies lateral rectus muscle)	**3**
d Complications ○ Globe perforation/rupture ○ Retrobulbar haemorrhage ○ Intravascular injection ○ Intrathecal injection ○ Injection into optic nerve ○ Failure	**6**
Reduce complication rate by: ○ Needle length ≤ 2.5 cm ○ Especial care or avoidance of block in high myopes with an axial globe length of ≥ 26 mm ○ Injection site to be within the infero-temporal quadrant	**3**

Question 3

What are the

a cardiovascular (25%),

b respiratory (25%),

c gastrointestinal (20%) and

d haematological (30%) potential benefits of local anaesthetic neuraxial blockade?

Curriculum reference: 13.1.5	
Answers	Marks for each (max)
a Cardiovascular ❍ Reduction of sympathetic activity leading to decreased incidence of: 1 Tachycardia 2 BP 3 Arrhythmias **(1 mark for each)** ❍ Reduced incidence of myocardial ischaemia/infarction. **(1)** ❍ Improved vascular graft patency. **(1)**	**5**
b Respiratory ❍ Improved pulmonary mechanics with effective pain relief allowing the patient to take a deep breath, cough and co-operate with physiotherapy. **(2)** ❍ Reduces the incidence of post-operative atelectasis and pulmonary infection and so improves post-operative oxygenation. **(2)** ❍ Avoidance of high-dose systemic opioids reduces respiratory depression and other effects of opioids. **(1)**	**5**
c Gastrointestinal ❍ Reducing systemic opioid use and improving intestinal motility by blocking nociceptive and sympathetic reflexes, reduces the duration of post-operative ileus and so permits earlier enteral feeding. **(3)** ❍ Bowel well contracted improving surgical operating conditions. **(1)**	**4**
d Haematological function/thromboembolic complications ❍ Intra-operative blood loss is reduced and so decreased requirements for blood products. **(2)** ❍ Attenuates the hypercoagulable response to surgery and improves fibrinolytic function. **(2)** ❍ Reduces the incidence of DVT and pulmonary thrombo-embolism. **(2)**	**6**

Question 4

a Describe the initial management options following a paracetamol overdose. (25%)

b What clinical features may develop following an untreated paracetamol overdose? (45%)

c List the biochemical and haematological abnormalities that may occur at 72 hours following an untreated paracetamol overdose. (30%)

Curriculum reference: 4.1.56 and 4.1.57	
Answers	Marks for each (max)
a Initial management ○ If < 1 hour since ingestion consider oral/NG activated charcoal/ gastric lavage ○ Take paracetamol levels at 4 hours post ingestion ○ Treat with iv N-acetylcysteine (NAC) ≤ 24 hrs post ingestion ○ NAC treatment guided by paracetamol concn/time since ingestion nomograms ○ Oral methionine therapy alternative antidote if IV treatment refused (but less effective than NAC)	**5**
b Clinical features ○ May be asymptomatic in first 24 hrs ○ Anorexia/ nausea and vomiting ○ Abdominal pain (right hypochondrium). ○ Hypoglycaemia causing decreased level of consciousness (↓LOC) ○ Hepatic encephalopathy – ↓LOC ○ Cerebral oedema – ↓LOC ○ Jaundice ○ Oliguria/loin pain/haematuria (incipient renal failure) ○ Hyperventilation (2° to metabolic acidosis) ○ Bleeding from IV cannulation sites (2° to coagulopathy)	**9**
c Blood test abnormalities ○ ↑ LFTs ○ ↑ Creatinine ○ ↑ Bilirubin ○ Metabolic acidosis – ↓ pH, ↑ H+, ↑ Lactate ○ ↓ Blood glucose ○ ↑ Prothrombin time (↑ INR)	**6**

Question 5

A two-year-old child presents to the Emergency Department (ED) with sudden onset of fever (38.5°C aural), sore throat, drooling and stridor.

a What conditions should be considered in the differential diagnosis? (25%)

b What would be your initial management of this child in the ED? (30%)

c How would you subsequently manage a deteriorating child? (45%)

Curriculum reference: 7.1.9, 10.1.2 and 10.1.4.

Answers	Marks for each (max)
a Differential diagnosis ❍ Acute epiglottitis ❍ Croup (acute tracheolaryngobronchitis) ❍ Inhaled foreign body ❍ Peritonsillar abscess (quinsy) ❍ Retropharyngeal abscess ❍ Bacterial tracheitis ❍ Diphtheria ❍ Glandular fever (infectious mononucleosis)	**5**
b Initial management ❍ Recognition of an emergency situation ❍ Commence non-threatening blow-by O_2 therapy ❍ Mobilise senior support (consultant anaesthetist and ENT surgeon) ❍ Inform operating theatres ❍ Avoid distressing the child (no oral examination, blood tests/ intravenous cannula, X-rays, forced O_2 therapy, parental separation) ❍ Do not leave child unattended ❍ Nebulised adrenaline	**6**
c Subsequent management ❍ Transfer to operating theatre/anaesthetic room ❍ Ensure ENT surgeon present for surgical airway if needed ❍ Gaseous induction ❍ Intubate under deep inhalational anaesthesia ❍ Swab for epiglottitis if indicated by laryngoscopy findings ❍ Oral followed by nasal tracheal tube ❍ IV access only after induction ❍ Take blood for FBC, blood cultures, biochemistry ❍ Commence broad spectrum IV antibiotics and steroids if indicated ❍ Sedate and continue IPPV/transfer to PICU/arrange retrieval	**9**

Question 6

a List the anaesthetic factors that predispose to peri-operative dental damage (25%).

b List the patient-related factors that predispose to peri-operative dental damage (25%)

c A 22-year-old man anaesthetised by a colleague awakens following tonsillectomy and complains that an upper incisor tooth has broken off during the operation. What is your management of this situation? (50%)

<table>
<tr><td colspan="2">Curriculum references: Professionalism III-6 and 1.1.83</td></tr>
<tr><td>Answers</td><td>Marks for each (max)</td></tr>
<tr><td>a Anaesthetic factors
○ Difficulty in maintaining airway/Difficulty with intubation (accept increasing Mallampati score)
○ Inexperienced anaesthetic personnel – operator technique (inexperienced anaesthetist)
○ Use of oral airway adjuncts – include airways, LMAs, bronchoscopes, airway instruments (Magills forceps), airway suction, etc
○ Laryngoscopy and tracheal intubation
○ Emergency anaesthesia, RSI, difficult access to patient
○ Emergence teeth clenching and inadequate depth of anaesthesia</td><td>5</td></tr>
<tr><td>b Patient-related factors
○ Patient characteristics: age (extremes of age), obesity, limited neck movement
○ Adverse oral anatomy: isolated, missing or abnormally positioned teeth, limited mandibular mobility, malocclusion (e.g. maxillary protrusion, overbite)
○ Dental pathology and drug therapy which is detrimental to optimal dental health: previous dental injury, caries, periodontal and gingival disease: drugs which reduce saliva production (e.g. anti-cholinergics,-psychotics etc); drugs in sugary vehicles (e.g. methodone); drugs which lower oral pH (e.g. inhaled asthma medication); drugs which cause gingival hypertrophy (e.g. phenytoin, nifedipine, cyclosporin, etc).
○ Previous restorative treatment: bridges, crowns, implants, braces
○ Systemic disease with oral manifestations: any disease which reduces saliva production or increases oral acid; smoking, diabetes, HIV, pregnancy, osteoporosis, blood dyscrasias, bulimia, gastro-oesophageal reflux</td><td>1 mark for each bold heading with example

Max 5</td></tr>
<tr><td colspan="2">answer continues/...</td></tr>
</table>

c Management of broken tooth ○ Apologise to patient ○ Discuss with senior colleague ○ Ensure colleague who anaesthetised patient is informed ○ Review pre-operative assessment of patient's dentition: Review anaesthetic chart/operating note for any mention of intra-operative dental damage ○ Examine the patient's mouth; ? extent of the dental damage; ? tooth present in mouth ○ If tooth found and avulsed whole seek urgent advice regarding possible re-implantation ○ Essential to exclude possibility that tooth has entered lower airway with CXR/CT scan ○ If any doubt that tooth is in the lower airway, rigid bronchoscopy for assessment/removal ○ Document your discussion with the patient and any management in the medical notes ○ Ensure incident form completed ±Trust risk manager contacted according to local guidelines ○ Discuss with patient arrangements for remedial dental treatment according to local protocols	**10**

Question 7

a What are i) diagnostic and ii) other clinical features of severe pre-eclampsia? (40%)

b What are the indications for magnesium therapy in severe pre-eclampsia/ eclampsia and which administration regimen(s) should be used? (20%)

c What are the symptoms and signs of magnesium toxicity (25%) and how should it be managed? (15%)

Curriculum reference: 6.1.9	
Answers	Marks for each (max)
a Diagnostic and clinical features of pre-eclampsia ***i) Diagnostic:*** Severe pre-eclampsia is severe hypertension with significant proteinuria, or moderate hypertension diastolic > 100 mm Hg and proteinuria and two other clinical features or HELLP ○ Severe Hypertension: Systolic BP > 160–170 mm Hg or diastolic > 110 mm Hg on two occasions **(1 mark with one value)** ○ Significant Proteinuria: > 1 g L^{-1} or 5 g/24 hr or > 3+ on dipstick **(1 mark)** ○ HELLP – haemolysis, ↑ elevated liver enzymes ↓ platelets **(1 mark)** ***ii) Other features*** ○ Renal: oliguria – < 400–500 ml/24 hrs (or less than 100 ml over a four hour period) or raised creatinine ○ Pulmonary oedema or respiratory compromise ○ CNS: headache, visual disturbance, clonus or convulsions ○ Epigastric pain (or right upper quadrant), liver rupture ○ Low platelet count: < 100 x 10^9 L^{-1} ○ Elevated liver enzymes: ALT or AST > 70 iu	**8**
b Magnesium therapy ○ In pre-eclampsia when there is concern about the risk of eclampsia ○ As therapy of choice for control of seizures ○ A loading dose of 4–5 g (16–20 mmol) by intravenous infusion over 5–10 minutes followed by maintenance infusion of 1 g hr^{-1} (4 mmoL hr^{-1}) until 24 hours after delivery or 24 hours after the last seizure **(2 marks for full answer)** ○ Recurrent seizures should be treated with a further 2 g (8 mmol) 'bolus' or an increase in infusion rate to 1.5 or 2.0 g hr^{-1} (6–8 mmol hr^{-1})	**4**
answer continues/...	

c Symptoms and signs ○ Nausea, vomiting ○ Somnolence, drowsiness (but not coma/unconsciousness) ○ Double vision ○ Slurred speech ○ Loss of deep tendon reflexes ○ Muscle weakness/paralysis ○ Cardiac or respiratory depression/arrest	**5**
Management ○ Reduce or stop infusion (**1 mark)** ○ Calcium chloride 1 g (10 ml 10% solution) IV over 10 minutes **(1 mark for dose and speed of infusion)** ○ Respiratory support/intubation/cardiovascular 'support'	**3**

Mg
Therapeutic – 2–4 mmol/L
loss of Reflex – 5 mmol/L
Resp rate ↓ – 6–7 mmol/L
Cardiac arrest – 12 mmol/L

SAQ **Answers**

Question 8

a What are the considerations when administering a general anaesthetic to a patient in the neuroradiology suite? (50%)

b List the common interventional neuroradiological procedures that may require general anaesthesia. (25%)

c Outline the possible complications of interventional neuroradiological procedures. (25%)

Curriculum references: In 5.2.27 and In 5.2.28	
Answers	Marks for each (max)
a Considerations ○ Possible remote site of INR suite ○ Poor lighting ○ Poor access to patient ○ Risk of exposure of radiation (radiation safety) ○ Transfer and medical management of critically ill patients to and from radiology suites ○ 'Neuroanaesthetic anaesthetic' technique. Avoid N_2O ○ May have to deliberately induce hypo or hypertension (arterial line monitoring essential) ○ Will need urinary catheter (significant infusion of flush and contrast media) ○ Smooth and rapid recovery from anaesthesia to facilitate early neurological assessment ○ Should be sufficient slack in tubing of lines and airways to allow safe movement ○ Prolonged procedures with potential for hypothermia ○ Careful management of anticoagulation is required to prevent thromboembolic complications during and after procedures.	**10**
b Common interventional procedures ○ Endovascular treatment of intracranial aneurysms ○ Embolisation of arteriovenous malformations ○ Tumour embolisation ○ Carotid stenosis angioplasty ○ Ischaemic stroke treatment ○ Trigeminal ganglion ablation	**5**
answer continues/...	

c Complications CNS complications: ❍ Haemorrhagic: Aneurysm perforation, intracranial vessel injury/ dissection ❍ Embolic: Thromboembolic complications, displacement of coil into parent vessel, coil fracture and vasospasm Non-CNS complications: ❍ Contrast reactions, contrast nephropathy ❍ Haemorrhage into puncture site/groin haematoma/ retroperitoneal haematoma/limb ischaemia	**5**

Question 9

a List the effects of physiological or excess cortisol that are of anaesthetic relevance. (40%)

b What are the causes of adrenocortical insufficiency? (30%)

c How may acute corticosteroid insufficiency be diagnosed clinically and biochemically? (30%)

Curriculum references: In 4.1.38 and In 22.1.9	
Answers	Marks for each (max)
a Effects ***Metabolic effects:*** ○ Stimulate gluconeogenesis and decrease cellular glucose/ anti-insulin causing hyperglycaemia ○ Mobilise amino acids and fatty acids/ ketogenesis ○ Protein catabolism/myopathy ○ Na and fluid retention/ hypertension ○ Hypokalaemia ***Other effects*** ○ ↑ RBC, neutrophil, and platelet levels ○ Exhibit anti-inflammatory effects ○ Maintenance of normal vascular response to vasoconstrictors ○ Immunodepression (especially lymphocytes) ○ Suppression of osteoblastic activity ○ Inhibition of collagen synthesis/ delayed wound healing	**8**
b Causes of adrenocortical insufficiency ○ ***Primary:*** Autoimmune atrophy, anatomical destruction by tumour and infection (TB/fungal infections), adrenal haemorrhage (sepsis or anticoagulation induced), congenital adrenal hyperplasia and drugs (e.g. metyrapone/cytotoxic agents, etomidate/ ketoconazole) ○ ***Secondary:*** Hypothalamic-pituitary disease (Sheehan's syndrome, trauma, cocaine abuse and SAH), HPA suppression by exogenous or endogenous steroids	**6**
answer continues/...	

c Clinical features ○ Fatigue or muscle weakness; postural hypotension/cardiovascular collapse; pigmentation ○ Evidence of septic shock and refractory hypotension despite resuscitation with fluids and vasopressors	**2**
Associated biochemical abnormalities: ○ Hypoglycaemia, hyponatraemia, hyperkalaemia and hypocalcaemia ○ Hyperprolactinaemia and hypothyroidism	**2**
Specific biochemical investigations: ○ ↓ random or basal plasma cortisol levels ○ Low or high dose short synthetic Tetracosactrin (synacthen) ACTH stimulation tests. 1 µg or 250 µg of synacthen given IV or IM. Blood samples taken for measurement of plasma cortisol levels at 30 minutes or at one hour. In healthy individuals the cortisol level should double within 60 minutes or increase to above 18 µg dl^{-1} (~500 nm L^{-1}) or an increase of ≥ 9 µg dl^{-1} (~250 nm L^{-1}).	**2**

Question 10

a How may a patient with sickle cell disease present in an acute crisis? (20%)

b Outline the important pre-operative (30%), intra-operative (35%) and post-operative (15%) considerations when anaesthetising a patient with sickle cell disease for an elective procedure.

Curriculum reference: In 21.1.9.	
Answers	Marks for each (max)
a Presentation in an acute crisis ○ Vaso-occlusive crisis – acute abdomen, 'acute chest syndrome', stroke, priapism, dactylitis ○ Aplastic crisis – precipitous fall in haemoglobin, absence of reticulocytes ○ Sequestration crisis (occurs mainly in children) – hypotension, severe anaemia ○ Haemolytic crisis – fall in haemoglobin, rise in reticulocytes and bilirubin	**4**
b Anaesthetic considerations ***Pre-operative assessment and preparation*** ○ Assess disease severity and organ function especially the cardio-respiratory systems ○ Minimise fasting period and ensure pre-operative hydration to prevent sickling (admit patients one day before surgery?) ○ Pre-operative investigations: chest X-ray, electrocardiogram, full blood count, urea and electrolytes, liver function tests and oxygen saturation ○ Consider pre-operative chest physiotherapy ○ Seek expert advice from haematologist ○ Consider transfusion to correct anaemia and/ or reduce HbS concentration	**6**
Intra-operative management ○ No evidence that any one anaesthetic technique is superior to another ○ Pre-oxygenate patient and avoid hypoxaemia throughout ○ Controlled ventilation is recommended to maintain normocarbia and avoid acidosis ○ Avoid dehydration and hypotension. Titrate induction agents carefully and replace fluid losses promptly ○ Monitor temperature and keep patient warm ○ Avoid use of epinephrine with local anaesthetic solutions ○ Use of tourniquet is extremely controversial. Meticulous exsanguination before inflation	**7**
Post-operative management ○ Recognise that most of the serious complications of sickle cell disease can occur in the post-operative period ○ Ensure oxygen supplementation, hydration, analgesia, normothermia ○ Lower threshold for HDU care ○ Day surgery may be inadvisable	**3**

Question 11

a Define the term 'inadvertent peri-operative hypothermia'. (10%)

b What are the physical mechanisms by which heat is lost from a patient in an operating theatre? (25%)

c List the clinical complications of hypothermia in the peri-operative period. (30%)

d Outline the current recommendations in the UK for the prevention of peri-operative hypothermia. (35%)

Curriculum references: In 14.1.6 and In 21.1.55.	
Answers	Marks for each (max)
a Definition The unintentional development of a core temperature of equal or less than 36°C in the peri-operative period (One hour before to 24 hours after surgery)	**2**
b Mechanisms ❍ Radiation (40%) ❍ Convection (30%) ❍ Evaporation (15%) ❍ Respiratory (10%) – 8% evaporation of water and 2% heating air ❍ Conduction (5%)	**5**
c Complications ❍ Shivering in recovery leading to increased oxygen consumption/ pain ❍ Greater blood loss in theatre and consequent need for blood transfusion ❍ Angina, myocardial infarction, ventricular tachycardia and cardiac arrest ❍ Increased incidence of wound infection ❍ Pressure sores ❍ Prolonged stay in recovery (in part due to impaired drug metabolism)	**6**
answer continues/...	

SAQ **Answers**

d Recommendations for prevention NICE (2008) ***Pre-operative:*** Risk assessment of patient. The patient is then given information on how to reduce their individual risk of hypothermia. Temperature should be measured in the hour prior to surgery. If < 36°C, then active warming established until normothermic.	**2**
Intra-operative: Forced air warming should be established as soon as possible (preferably in the anaesthetic room) for any patient having an anaesthetic time of > 30 minutes or has two or more risk factors for inadvertent peri-operative hypothermia. Intravenous fluids should be warmed. Core temperature to be measured and recorded every 30 minutes.	**3**
Post-operative: Patients should not be discharged from recovery until their temperature reaches 36°C. The temperature should be recorded with the same frequency as the other standard post-operative investigations for 24 hours (inpatients).	**2**

Question 12

a A 24-year-old male is scheduled for exploration and laying open of a pilonidal sinus under general anaesthesia. Outline the anaesthetic implications of managing this patient in the prone position. (45%)

b How may the complications of this position be minimised? (55%)

Curriculum reference: 12.1.7	
Answers	Marks for each (max)
a Anaesthetic implications	
Technical: Adequate personnel to turn from supine to prone position. Potential for IV line to be pulled out, monitoring wires and tubes becoming disconnected or trapped under the patient.	**2**
Airway/Respiratory: Airway obstruction; accidental extubation; endobronchial intubation; reduced chest wall compliance/splinting of diaphragm leading to hypoxia and raised airway pressures.	**2**
Cardiovascular: Reduced CO/ hypotension (IVC compression); femoral artery compression (vascular insufficiency).	**1**
Ophthalmic: Corneal abrasions; raised intraocular pressure.	**1**
Neurological: Peripheral nerve injuries (brachial plexus, femoral, supraorbital and lateral cutaneous nerve of the thigh).	**1**
Musculoskeletal: Backache, hyperextension injury to cervical spine and shoulder dislocation.	**1**
Cutaneous: Pressure damage to skin of feet, knees, anterior superior iliac spine and tip of nose.	**1**
b Minimising complications related to prone position	
Avoid the prone position and anaesthetise the patient in the lateral position. When turning to prone position temporarily disconnect the IV line and the monitoring tubes/wires.	**2**
Airway/Respiratory: Intubated and ventilated with cuffed armoured tracheal tube. Particular attention paid to securing the tube to the face (? Tape <u>and</u> tie). Disconnect tube from breathing circuit when the patient is turned into the prone position and then the chest auscultated to exclude tube migration.	**2**
Cardiovascular: Large bore intravenous access and avoid abdominal compression using a specialised mattress. Once positioned in the prone position, check the peripheral pulses.	**2**
Ophthalmic: Tape and pad the eyes and avoid direct pressure on them (particularly if the patient has glaucoma).	**1**
Neurological: Take care to avoid stretching brachial plexus or direct pressure on the peripheral nerves.	**1**
Musculoskeletal: Avoid hyperextension of neck, position the face on a soft pillow or other support with the neck comfortably flexed and rotated. Controlled log-roll with the limbs in a neutral position.	**2**
Cutaneous: Adequate padding of pressure points.	**1**

SAQ Paper 2

Question 1

a How may pain following Caesarean section (CS) performed under general anaesthesia be managed? (35%)

b What neuraxial techniques may be used to provide post-operative analgesia following CS? (Include appropriate dose ranges). (20%)

c What are the monitoring requirements after CS following spinal or epidural opioid administration? (15%)

d List the side effects of neuraxially administered opioids and how may these be managed? (30%)

Curriculum reference: 8.1.5 ; 8.1.7; 8.1.10	
Answers	Marks to total of 20
a Analgesia following general anaesthesia for Caesarean section ***Simple analgesia:*** ○ Paracetamol 1 gm 6-hourly ○ Diclofenac 50 mg 8-hourly (if no contraindication) for all patients **(max 2 points)** ***Opiates:*** ○ IV morphine during CS ○ PCA morphine for first 24 hours, followed after 24 hours by ○ Tramadol 50–100 mg 8 hourly (manufacturers caution in breast-feeding) ○ Codeine 30–60 mg 6 hourly ○ Oramorph 10–20 mg 2 hourly **(max 3 points)** ***Regional/LA:*** ○ Bilateral ilioinguinal nerve blocks ○ Bilateral transversus abdominis plane (TAP) blocks ○ Wound infiltration with 20 ml levo-bupivacaine 0.5% **(max 2 points)**	**7**
b Neuraxial techniques ***Spinal:*** Long acting intrathecal opiates (NOT fentanyl) Preservative free morphine 75–200 µg; or diamorphine 200–500 µg; clonidine 75–150 µg ***Epidural:*** Diamorphine 2.5–3 mg or preservative free morphine 3–4 mg; Clonidine 150–600 µg or PCEA/infusion of opiate and local anaesthetic mixture	**4**
answer continues/...	

c Monitoring Basic monitoring (Resp rate/sedation score/pulse/BP/SaO_2) Timing (every 30 min for two hours and two hourly for 24 hours) Modified Early Obstetric Warning Scoring (MEOWS) chart	**Max 3**
d Side effects ❍ Sedation – close observation required ❍ Respiratory depression – treat with high dose naloxone 400 μg ❍ Nausea and vomiting – treat with intravenous cyclizine 50 mg IV eight hourly (safe in breast-feeding) or ondansetron ❍ Pruritus – treat with incremental doses of naloxone, antihistamines, 5-HT_3 antagonists (e.g. ondansetron), droperidol 1–2.5 mg, incremental propofol ❍ Constipation – manage with lactulose or senna ❍ Urinary retention – bladder care/monitoring and early catheterisation ❍ Delayed gastric emptying – appropriate gastric prokinetic	**Max 6**

Question 2

a What are the central and peripheral neurological complications of coronary artery bypass (CABG) surgery? (35%)

b What are the risk factors for central neurological complications following CABG surgery? (30%)

c How can the risk of central neurological complications of CABG surgery be reduced? (35%)

Curriculum reference: 9.1.4; 9.1.5	
Answers	Marks to total of 20
a Major neurological complications ○ ***Brain:* (max 4 marks)** Cognitive impairment Altered level of consciousness (delirium, coma) visual field defects Stroke – thromboembolic, haemorrhagic, ischaemic Seizures – particularly in children Emergence of primitive reflexes ○ ***Spinal cord:*** Ischaemia/paraplegia **(max 1 mark)** ○ ***Nerve plexuses:* (max 2 marks)** Brachial plexus injury – excessive use of sternal retractor Peripheral nerve injury – ulnar neuropathy – incorrect positioning	**7**
b Risk factors ***Patient factors*** ○ Atheroma of the proximal aorta ○ History of neurological injury (i.e. stroke/TIA) ○ Diabetes mellitus ○ Old age, hypertension, lung disease ***Surgical factors*** ○ Cardiopulmonary bypass ○ Previous surgery ○ Use of intra aortic balloon pump ○ Tranexamic acid	**6**
answer continues/...	

c Reducing risk ❍ Modify technique – avoid multiple aortic cross-clamping ❍ Image proximal aorta – TOE or epiaortic ultrasound ❍ Modify bypass Minimise exposure to bypass Maintain pressure and flow Avoid air entrainment Use membrane oxygenator/arterial line filter Avoid hyperthermia during rewarming Maintain glucose control ❍ Use neurological monitoring – TCD, NIRS, EEG ❍ Pharmacological neuroprotection – propofol, steroids, NMDA antagonists, lidocaine, magnesium, barbiturates	**7**

Question 3

A 67-year-old man requires a thoraco-abdominal oesophagectomy for adenocarcinoma.

a Describe the clinical features associated with the condition that are relevant to anaesthesia. (35%)

b List the pre-operative investigations you might need to consider. (30%)

c What aspects of peri-operative anaesthetic care can help reduce post-operative morbidity following this procedure? (35%)

Curriculum reference: 3.2.12; 9.1.19; 9.1.25; B1.2.54; B1.2.55	
Answers	Marks to total of 20
a Relevant clinical features ***General issues:*** ❍ Oesophageal obstruction and dysphagia ❍ Gastro-oesophageal reflux and pulmonary aspiration ❍ Nutritional status, loss of weight, electrolyte imbalance and anaemia. ❍ Immunosuppression from chemotherapy/radiotherapy ***Cardiopulmonary disease:*** ❍ Smoking and alcohol use ❍ High incidence of IHD and hypertension ❍ COPD	**7**
b Pre-operative investigations ❍ Routine biochemistry, haematology, clotting screen, group and cross match **(1 mark)** ❍ Twelve lead ECG/transthoracic echo **(1 mark)** ❍ Pulmonary function tests including gas transfer (DLCO/KCO), FEV1, FEV1/FVC, VC **(1 mark)** ❍ Baseline arterial blood gases on room air **(1 mark)** ❍ Chest X-ray **(1 mark)** ❍ Cardiopulmonary exercise testing (CPX)/coronary angiography/cardiac stress testing **(1 mark)**	**6**
c Morbidity reduction ❍ Respiratory optimisation ❍ Use of a thoracic epidural ❍ Goal-directed fluid management therapy ❍ Protective ventilation during one-lung anaesthesia ❍ Strategies to improve perfusion of the gastric graft ❍ Maintain normothermia ❍ Adequate nutrition	**7**

BCIS ✓

Question 4

a Describe the anatomy of the cervical plexus. (40%)

b How would you perform a superficial cervical plexus block? (25%)

c A carotid endarterectomy is being performed using a superficial cervical plexus block. A few minutes after clamping the carotid artery the patient becomes unresponsive to verbal command. Describe your management of this situation. (35%)

Curriculum reference: 13.2.15; 20.1.5	
Answers	Marks to total of 20
a Anatomy of the cervical plexus ***Anterior rami of C1–C4 form 3 loops, from which arise:*** ❍ Communicating branches from cervical plexus to hypoglossal n (from C1), to ansa hypoglossi (C2) and phrenic (C3 and C4)	**2**
Deep cervical plexus: branches to anterior vertebral muscles, and contributes to innervation of scalenus medius, sternomastoid and trapezius muscles.	**2**
Superficial cervical plexus: Four branches, supply skin of the neck: 1. Lesser occipital (C2) 2. Great auricular (C2 and C3) 3. Anterior cutaneous nerve of the neck (C2 and C3) 4. Supraclavicular (C3 and C4) Plexus lies on scalenus medius behind sternomastoid, superficial branches loop around the middle portion of sternomastoid.	**4**
b Cervical plexus block How would you perform a superficial cervical plexus block? Usual precautions – IV access, trained assistant, asepsis, resuscitation capability. 5–10 ml of LA injected at posterior border of mid-point of sternomastoid muscle, in a 'fan' or 'sausage' pattern.	**Max 5**
c Unresponsive patient ❍ Tell the surgeon ❍ Airway – bag/mask initially ❍ Breathing – give 100% oxygen (may improve neurology), IPPV if required ❍ Circulation – increase BP to at least normal for that patient ❍ Ask surgeon to unclamp carotid and consider inserting a shunt ❍ GA – ▪ maintains airway (LMA or ETT) and oxygenation ▪ access difficult ▪ avoid hypotension ▪ may be neuroprotective	**Max 7**

SAQ **Answers**

Question 5

A 30-year-old man attempted suicide by jumping from a building. He sustained severe trauma including major facial injuries.

a What are the potential airway management problems? (25%)

b List five possible options for securing the airway in this patient. (25%)

c Outline the potential disadvantages for each of these options? (50%)

Curriculum reference: 16.1.6	
Answers	Marks to total of 20
a Airway problems ○ Disruption of bony structures and soft tissues ○ Swelling of the airway ○ Blood, secretions and foreign bodies in the airway ○ Potential C-spine injury and neck immobilisation ○ Loss of airway/risk of aspiration if conscious level reduced	**5**
b Options of securing airway ○ Rapid sequence induction and intubation ○ Awake tracheostomy/cricothyroidotomy ○ Inhalational induction and intubation ○ Awake fibreoptic intubation ○ Retrograde intubation ○ Supraglottic devices	**Max 5**
c Disadvantages ***General*** Need patient co-operation Risk of aspiration Loss of airway and 'can't intubate can't ventilate' scenario C-Spine injury ***RSI*** ○ Manual inline mobilisation/cricoid pressure may complicate intubation ○ Hypotension due to induction agents possible ○ May be difficult to do effective pre-oxygenation ***Awake tracheostomy/cricothyroidotomy*** ○ May be difficult technically in presence of injury ***Inhalational induction*** ○ Difficult to get good seal with facial injury ○ Slow induction ○ Possibility of airway obstruction – oedema and blood ***Awake fibreoptic intubation*** ○ Poor image due to blood and secretions ○ Local anaesthesia of airway inadequate ○ Fibreoptic endoscopy technically difficult with abnormal anatomy ***Retrograde intubation*** – appropriate equipment required ***Supraglottic device*** – does not secure airway	**Max 10**

Question 6

a List the complications associated with the delivery of high partial pressures of oxygen? (60%)

b What are the oxygen saturation targets of oxygen therapy in: (i) previously healthy adult patients and (ii) patients with chronic obstructive pulmonary disease (COPD)? (10%)

c What are the postulated cellular mechanisms of oxygen toxicity? (10%)

d Which common themes associated with oxygen therapy were identified by the National Patient Safety Agency (NPSA) in 2009 as having contributed to patient deaths? (20%)

Curriculum reference: 10.2.18	
Answers	Marks to total of 20
a Respiratory system	
Acute: Hypoventilation (patients with chronically raised $PaCO_2$ and an established hypoxic drive), tracheobronchitis and absorption atelectasis (symptoms include sub-sternal heaviness, pleuritic chest pain, cough and dyspnoea. Chronic: Interstitial pulmonary fibrosis. Bronchopulmonary dysplasia in neonates.	**5**
Central nervous system: Acute: High concentrations of oxygen administered in a hyperbaric chamber may cause perioral tingling, irritability, tinnitus, nausea, altered behaviour and seizures. Neurogenic pulmonary oedema has also been described.	**2**
Ophthalmic system: Reversible constriction of peripheral vision progressive myopia, cataract formation and retrolental fibroplasia (associated with premature infants).	**2**
Cardiovascular system: May increase infarct size in 'uncomplicated' myocardial infarction.	**1**
Other – explosion and fire risks – humidification issues	**2**
b Saturation targets (i) Previously healthy patients 94–98% (ii) COPD – 88–92%	**2**
c Cellular mechanisms ***Free radicals production:*** superoxide anion (O_2^-), hydroxyl radical and hydrogen peroxide cause: ○ Lipid peroxidation ○ Inhibit nucleic acids and protein synthesis ○ Inactivation of cellular enzymes Normally antioxidant enzymes (glutathione peroxidase, catalase and superoxide dismutase) donate electrons to scavenge and neutralise the free radicals. ***Non-radical mediated injury:*** Inhibition of glutamic acid decarboxylase and reduce GABA in CNS may contribute to seizures.	**2**
answer continues/...	

d NPSA themes ***Prescribing:*** Failure to prescribe or incorrect dosage used. ***Monitoring:*** Patients not monitored; recognised hypoxia not dealt with. ***Administration:*** Confusion between compressed air and oxygen. Incorrect flow rates and inadvertent disconnection of supply. ***Equipment:*** Empty cylinders; faulty and missing equipment.	**4**

Question 7

a Describe the three essential stages of the World Health Organization (WHO) safety checklist and when should they occur in relation to each operative procedure? (15%)

b What information needs to be exchanged between the anaesthetic, surgical and theatre teams as part of the checklist? (70%)

c Which aspects of the checklist are designed to decrease surgical site infection? (15%)

Curriculum reference: In: 1.1.2; In: 1.1.5; Professionalism III-6	
Answers	Marks to total of 20
a Three stages ❍ Sign in – occurs before anaesthetic induction ❍ Time out – before surgery commences ❍ Sign out – at end of surgery	**3**
b Information exchange ❍ Team member introductions ❍ Correct identification of the patient ❍ Patient's ASA grade ❍ Anaesthetic monitoring equipment requirements ❍ Need for blood products ❍ Need for VTE prophylaxis ❍ Potential difficult airway/aspiration risk ❍ Anaesthetic machine check completed ❍ Any known allergies ❍ Adequate vascular access in place (if ↑ blood loss anticipated) ❍ Post-operative care issues/need for ICU etc ❍ Any other specific anaesthetic related issues (e.g. MH risk) ❍ Critical/unexpected steps during surgery ❍ Confirmation and marking of correct site/side ❍ Anticipated blood loss ❍ Specific surgical equipment or prostheses requirements ❍ Access to radiological investigations ❍ Special intra-operative investigations (e.g. X-ray screening)	**14**
c Surgical site infection checklist ❍ Need for antibiotic prophylaxis ❍ Need for patient warming ❍ Need for hair removal from surgical site ❍ Need for glycaemic control	**3**

Question 8

a List the modes of non-invasive respiratory support (NIRS). (20%)

b In what adult clinical scenarios may NIRS be indicated? (30%)

c What are the contraindications to NIRS? (30%)

d Summarise the clinical advantages of NIRS compared to conventional positive pressure ventilation via a tracheal tube. (20%)

Curriculum reference: In: 4.1.23	
Answers	Marks to total of 20
a Modes of non-invasive respiratory support ○ CPAP ○ Pressure assist (e.g. BiPAP) ○ Volume assist ○ Negative pressure ventilation	**4**
b Indications ○ Exacerbation of COPD/asthma ○ Pulmonary oedema ○ Hypoxaemia associated with pneumonia, chest trauma, early ARDS ○ Obesity and obstructive sleep apnoea ○ Weaning from conventional ventilation – bridge to prevent re-intubation ○ Respiratory failure in 'not for IPPV' situations (i.e. haematological malignancy and immunosuppressed patients) (e.g. chemotherapy effects, post-transplantation, AIDS) ○ Long-term ventilation for progressive neuromuscular disease/ spinal injuries	**6**
c Contraindications ○ Respiratory arrest (i.e. resuscitation mandates intubation) ○ Impaired level of consciousness ○ Bulbar palsy (aspiration risk) ○ Non-compliant patient ○ Recent facial surgery, facial deformity/ trauma/ burns ○ Recent upper GI surgery (anastomotic viability/ tension) ○ Inability to clear secretions	**6**
d Advantages ○ Avoids technical problems of tracheal intubation/extubation ○ Avoids problems due to presence of ETT and IPPV – ventilator associated pneumonia, ↓ ciliary function, sinusitis, endobronchial intubation, baro/volume trauma, inability to talk/eat, CVS instability ○ ↓ sedation requirement – CVS instability, weaning delay, impaired cough reflex, reduced GI motility ○ Other benefits: use in non-intensive care environments including domiciliary use	**4**

Question 9

a List the harmful chemicals in tobacco smoke. (15%)

b What are the pathophysiological effects of tobacco smoking on the cardiovascular (20%), respiratory (25%) and other body systems? (20%)

c What advice would you give to a smoker attending a pre-operative assessment clinic six weeks before a scheduled procedure under general anaesthesia? (20%)

Curriculum reference: In: 1.1.13; In: 20.1.11	
Answers	Marks to total of 20
a Harmful chemicals ❍ Nicotine, carbon monoxide, nitric oxide, hydrogen cyanide, tar and aldehydes	**3**
b Indications ***Cardiac:*** ❍ Nicotine: increased heart rate, SVR and blood pressure. Indirectly contributing to myocardial ischaemia ❍ Carbon monoxide: Negative inotrope. Myocardial ischaemia (coronary vasoconstriction, reduced oxygen carrying capacity) ❍ Arrhythmias with exercise ❍ Ischaemic heart disease, peripheral vascular disease, coronary vasospasm	**4**
Respiratory: ❍ Carbon monoxide increases the carboxyhaemoglobin levels: > 2–15%. ❍ Oxyhaemoglobin dissociation curve shifted to the left resulting in a decrease in oxygen supply ❍ Increase in mucus production, reduction in ciliary activity and impaired ability to clear secretions. Increased post-operative pulmonary complications (e.g. chest infection) ❍ Increased cough and bronchial reactivity results in increased likelihood of breath-holding, laryngo- and broncho-spasm at induction and recovery ❍ Decreased surfactant production, reduced lung compliance, closure of small airways ❍ COPD, emphysema, lung cancer	**5**
Other: ❍ **Immunological**: Immunosuppression resulting in increased chest and wound infections and delayed wound healing ❍ **Hepatic**: Enzymes induction resulting in higher doses required of some drugs ❍ **Neurological**: CNS stimulation and dependence ❍ Reduced incidence of PONV	**4**
answer continues/...	

c Advice ❍ Ideally avoid smoking for 12 hours pre-op: COHb T1/2 four hours and nicotine T1/2 30–60 mins. Minimum abstention for few hours useful. ❍ Need to stop smoking completely for as long as possible before surgery to reduce post-operative pulmonary complications (no evidence of harm from brief pre-operative abstinence). Patient should be aware that increased sputum production may occur in the initial period. ❍ Risk of wound infection changes to the same as for a non-smoker after four weeks so cessation for four weeks pre-operatively ideal. ❍ Should use pre-operative clinic as a 'teachable moment' to encourage permanent cessation, including providing advice as to how to stop (e.g. referral to national stop smoking helpline and leaflet distribution). Nicotine replacement therapy should be encouraged, but avoided immediately pre-operatively due to potential CVS effects.	**4**

Question 10

a What are the potential benefits of an enhanced recovery ('fast-track') programme for a patient undergoing major abdominal surgery? (25%)

b List the pre-operative (25%), intra-operative (25%) and post-operative goals (25%) that aim to achieve 'fast track' status.

Curriculum reference: In: 11.1.2	
Answers	Marks to total of 20
a Potential benefits ❍ Early recovery of bowel function/decreased duration of ileus ❍ Decreased post-operative complications, especially cardiopulmonary ❍ Decreased length of hospital stay, increased efficiency ❍ Increased muscle strength and exercise capacity ❍ Streamlines patient pathway and processes	**5**
b Fast track goals	
Pre-operative: ❍ Appropriate patient selection ❍ Patient education and motivation ❍ Pre-operative optimisation of co-morbidities ❍ Use of carbohydrate loading (clear complex carbohydrate drinks) ❍ Clear fluids up to two hours pre-operatively ❍ Avoidance of bowel preparation ❍ Avoidance of routine premedication	**5**
Intra-operative ❍ Surgical technique: transverse incision; minilaparotomy incision; laparoscopic technique ❍ Avoidance of routine nasogastric tubes and drains ❍ Fluid management: minimise use of crystalloids and targeted fluid replacement ❍ Use of quick offset anaesthetic agents to allow rapid recovery ❍ Opioid sparing analgesic technique (e.g. epidural analgesia, nerve blocks) ❍ Maintenance of normothermia ❍ Prevention of PONV (e.g. avoidance of nitrous oxide, use of TIVA and routine) ❍ Use of antiemetics	**5**
Post-operative ❍ Use of multimodal analgesia ❍ Encourage oral fluids early and early nutrition (energy drinks) ❍ Early mobilisation ❍ Prokinetics (e.g. metoclopramide) ❍ Minimisation of opioid usage ❍ Community support, helpline	**5**

Question 11

a What are the diagnostic (25%) and therapeutic (25%) indications for bronchoscopy?

b List the major contraindications for bronchoscopy. (20%)

c How should a fibreoptic bronchoscope be reprocessed after use? (30%)

Curriculum reference: 1.1.3; 1.2.9; 1.1.71; 9.1.21; 10.1.4	
Answers	Marks to total of 20
a Indicators ***Diagnostic*** ○ Investigation of respiratory disease ○ Bronchoalveolar lavage (BAL) ○ Tissue diagnosis and staging of tumours ○ Assess extent of airway injury (burns/trauma) ○ Assessment of endotracheal tube position (i.e. double lumen tube/percutaneous tracheostomy)	**5**
Therapeutic ○ Removal of a foreign body: Usually using a rigid scope under general anaesthesia ○ Removal of secretions which may be causing collapse/ consolidation of lung lobes ○ Respiratory toilet ○ Facilitate tracheal intubation ○ Tracheal surgery (laser surgery, tracheal dilatation)	**5**
b Major contraindications ○ Patient refusal ○ Unstable haemodynamic status/ life-threatening arrhythmias ○ Coagulopathy or bleeding diathesis that cannot be corrected ○ Inadequate facilities and experienced personnel to deal with the procedure ○ Failure to maintain oxygenation	**4**
c Decontamination procedures ○ Inspect external surface of the bronchoscope for damage and leak test ○ Wipe external surfaces and thoroughly brush and flush all internal channels with detergent ○ Disinfect with an agent of sufficient microbiological intensity at an adequate temperature and sufficient duration ○ Rinse thoroughly with filtered tap water followed by 70% ethyl alcohol or sterile water ○ Allow bronchoscope to dry thoroughly in a designated area ○ Store bronchoscope in a hanging position to prevent moisture accumulation ○ Traceability, tracking audit systems should be in place to ensure effective decontamination procedures and prevent cross infection	**6**

Question 12

You are asked to assess a 4-year-old child who is scheduled for a strabismus (squint) correction as a day case procedure.

a List the anaesthetic-related issues this case presents. (60%)

b During surgical traction, the patient suddenly develops a profound sinus bradycardia. How would you manage this situation? (10%)

c Describe the key post-operative problems and relevant management strategies. (30%)

Curriculum reference: 17.1.3; 17.2.3	
Answers	Marks to total of 20
a Anaesthetic issues ***Paediatric patient:*** ❍ Altered physiology and anatomy ❍ Altered psychology ❍ Paediatric trained staff/ unit ❍ Consent	**3**
Fulfil appropriate day case criteria: ❍ Anaesthetic/ surgical factors (relatively short surgery, no significant haemorrhage, not difficult airway) ❍ Medical factors (ASA1/2) ❍ Social factors (parent willing, not single carer with multiple other siblings, phone access, transport)	**3**
Problems of all ophthalmic surgery ❍ Limited access to the airway during surgery	**1**
Problems specific to squint surgery ❍ High incidence PONV ❍ Oculo-cardiac reflex (OCR) during surgery ❍ Significant post-operative pain	**3**
Miscellaneous ❍ Increased incidence of squint in children with underlying primary or secondary myopathy ❍ Malignant hyperpyrexia = contentious	**2**
b Bradycardia ❍ Ask surgeon to stop retracting ❍ Administer IV atropine or glycopyrrolate ❍ Exclude other causes (i.e. hypoxia)	**2**
answer continues/...	

c Post-operative problems ***PONV reduced by:*** ○ Avoiding prolonged fasting times ○ Intra-operative fluid administration ○ Using a TIVA technique ○ Avoiding opioids if possible ○ Combination anti-emetics; ondansetron (0.1 mg/kg^{-1}) and dexamethasone (0.1–0.2 $mg\ kg^{-1}$)	**3**
Post-operative pain management: ○ Multimodal approach with post-operative instructions ○ Regular oral paracetamol and NSAIDs ○ Amethocaine eye drops ○ Diclofenac eye drops + Sub-Tenon's ○ Other LA blocks	**3**

SAQ **Answers**

DIVINUM SEDARE DOLOREM

MCQ examination Multiple True or False (MTF)

No explanation will be given for true answers if they are self-explanatory.

1 The following are indications for pre-operative measurement of serum urea and electrolytes in patients admitted for elective surgery:

✓
✓
✓
✓
✗

Digoxin toxicity is enhanced by hypokalaemia. Diuretic therapy causes hypokalaemia. Insulin dependent diabetics and patients with recurrent urinary tract infections are prone to disturbances of serum urea and electrolytes. In the absence of a specific indication it is not appropriate to perform this investigation just because the patient is over 50 years old.

2 Hazards of anaesthesia in a patient with chronic renal failure include:

✓
✓
✓
✗
✓

Hypertension and pericarditis are complications of chronic renal failure. Left ventricular enlargement is associated with hypertension. Cardiac tamponade may result from a pericardial effusion or haemorrhage into the pericardium.

3 Hypophysectomy may result in:

✓
✗
✓
✓
✗

After hypophysectomy secretion of TSH and ACTH may cease, resulting in atrophy of the thyroid and the adrenal cortex. Diabetes insipidus does occur but is rare after hypophysectomy because the hypothalamus usually continues to secrete ADH bypassing the posterior pituitary.

4 **The following groups of people have an increased risk of latex allergy:**

✓ ✗ ✓ ✗ ✓

Health workers and those who have repeated surgical procedures have a greater response to latex. There is cross reactivity between some fruits (kiwi fruit, avocados and bananas) and latex. There is no greater risk in patients with penicillin allergy. Disposable tracheal tubes do not contain latex.

5 **Myocardial stunning:**

✗ ✗ ✓ ✗ ✓

Myocardial stunning is reversible, does not always follow myocardial ischaemia, and is not a cause of beta adrenoceptor down-regulation.

6 **Supraclavicular brachial plexus block differs from axillary brachial plexus block because the supraclavicular block:**

✗ ✗ ✓ ✓ ✗

Axillary brachial plexus block is less likely than supraclavicular block to provide analgesia for the lateral part of the forearm and more likely to involve intravascular injection of local anaesthetic. Both blocks will involve nerves to the intraosseous muscles to a similar extent.

7 **Severe middle third fractures of the face:**

✓ ✓ ✗ ✗ ✓

Any severe blow to the head can cause brain injury. Fractures to the face can obstruct the airway and cause bleeding into the airway. Fixation can wait for several days in the absence of continuing haemorrhage and obstruction of the airway. The patient does not require nasal intubation which may be harmful if there is a base of skull fracture.

8 **Phantom limb pain:**

✓ ✗ ✗ ✓ ✗

Motor nerves make no contribution to phantom limb pain. It is associated with pre-operative pain, but evidence for this may be questioned now. Phantom limb pain occurs after traumatic amputation of a limb.

9 Pain during the first stage of labour may be relieved by:

✓ ✓ ✗ ✗ ✓

A, B and E are true because pain during the first stage of labour is transmitted centrally with T11, T12 and L1 sympathetic nerves. Pudendal nerve block provides perineal analgesia only. Paracervical block only relieves pain associated with dilation of the cervix.

10 Symptoms or signs characteristic of amniotic fluid embolism include:

✓ ✓ ✓ ✗ ✗

Amniotic fluid embolism causes DIC and consumption of fibrin. Pulmonary embolism causes chest pain. The patient will be hypoxic and will hyperventilate. Hypotension is likely because of reduced delivery of blood to the left side of the heart.

11 At a core temperature of 30°C:

✓ ✗ ✗ ✗ ✓

Blood coagulability is decreased during hypothermia. Glomerular filtration is reduced but does not cease. Blood viscosity increases on cooling.

12 In a patient with porphyria:

✓ ✗ ✓ ✗ ✓

Dysautonomia is a feature of porphyric crisis. Glycine is safe and fluid restriction has no effect.

13 In myotonic dystrophy, spasticity of muscles is relieved by:

✗ ✗ ✗ ✓ ✗

Succinylcholine and neostigmine cause muscle spasticity in myotonic dystrophy. Spinal anaesthesia and dantrolene have no effect on spasticity.

14 Cardioversion is indicated in the treatment of:

✗
✓
✗
✓
✗

Sinus tachycardia can be slowed by carotid sinus massage and beta-blockers. Cardioversion will not help and may cause harm in junctional bradycardia or electro-mechanical dissociation.

15 Circulatory assistance by intra-aortic balloon pumping is useful because it:

✓
✗
✓
✗
✗

The balloon inflates in diastole raising aortic diastolic pressure and deflates in systole reducing afterload and myocardial work. It will tend to reduce aortic systolic pressure and reduce or have no effect on left atrial pressure and left ventricular end-diastolic pressure.

16 During storage of whole blood, the decrease in 2,3-diphosphoglycerate (2,3-DPG) concentration can be reduced by the addition of:

✗
✓
✗
✓
✓

Mannitol helps to prevent oxidative damage to RBC in storage and has no effect on 2,3-DPG. Pyruvate does not have an important role in blood storage.

17 In a sacral epidural (caudal) block in adults:

✓
✗
✗
✓
✓

The sacral hiatus and the posterior superior iliac spines form an equilateral triangle. The dura normally ends at S2. The pressure in the sacral canal is not negative. If the needle is subcutaneous the injection of air will cause palpable subcutaneous emphysema.

18 Structures supplied by segment S2 include the:

✗
✓
✓
✓
✓

The skin of the buttock is supplied by the posterior rami of S3, 4, 5.

19 Interruption of the cervical sympathetic chain results in:

✗ ✗ ✓ ✗ ✓

Interruption of the cervical sympathetic chain will cause constriction of the pupil. Taste sensation of the anterior two-thirds of the tongue is supplied by the facial nerve via the chorda tympani. Salivation is controlled by parasympathetic nerves.

20 The following agents may cause pulmonary fibrosis:

✓ ✗ ✓ ✓ ✗

Cortisone and organophosphate compounds do not cause pulmonary fibrosis.

21 Heat and moisture exchange filters:

✓ ✗ ✓ ✓ ✓

Heat moisture exchange filters should have a high thermal capacity and low thermal conductivity to retain heat for efficient revaporisation of the condensed water. They are less efficient as minute volume increases. They should filter out bacteria.

22 An abnormal response to suxamethonium occurs in patients suffering from:

✗ ✓ ✓ ✓ ✓

In dermatomyositis and dystrophia myotonica a dangerous increase in serum potassium occurs following suxamethonium. In hepatic failure suxamethonium is metabolised more slowly because of lower pseudocholinesterase levels. Collagen diseases cause a reduction in plasma cholinesterase levels.

23 The ventilatory response to hypoxia is decreased in patients:

✓ ✓ ✓ ✗ ✓

Peripheral chemoreceptors mediate this response and are depressed by anaesthesia and opioids. Acclimatisation to altitude resets this reflex. The reflex is also reset in patients with cyanotic congenital heart disease. Patients with pulmonary fibrosis have a normal ventilatory response to hypoxia and hyperventilate.

24 **The following drugs alter the level of thyroxine production:**

✓
✓
✗
✗
✗

Propranolol is useful to slow the heart rate in thyrotoxicosis but does not reduce thyroxine levels. Carbidopa is used in the treatment of Parkinson's disease. Prazocin is an alpha adrenergic blocking agent. Amiodarone contains iodine and modifies thyroxine production.

25 **Stimulation of postganglionic thoraco-lumbar autonomic nerve fibres produces:**

✓
✗
✓
✗
✗

The postganglionic thoraco-lumbar autonomic nerve fibres are sympathetic and cause bronchodilation, an increase in myocardial rhythmicity and an increase in myocardial contractility.

26 **The alveolar-arterial oxygen tension difference is increased by:**

✓
✗
✓
✓
✓

Nitrous oxide uptake by the concentration effect will increase alveolar oxygen concentrations but only in perfused alveoli so the alveolar–arterial oxygen difference will not increase. Ventilation/perfusion mismatch increases the differences and a reduction in FRC and hepatic failure increases V/Q mismatch.

27 **Pulmonary vascular resistance is reduced by:**

✗
✗
✓
✓
✓

Hypoxic pulmonary vasoconstriction raises pulmonary vascular resistance. Alkalosis in the pulmonary vascular bed mimics the effect of acidosis in the systemic capillaries. Nitric oxide and prostacyclin have a direct effect on the vascular smooth muscle.

28 **Complement is required for:**

✓
✗
✗
✓
✗

Complement proteins are activated classically by antigen-antibody combinations and are bound by IgG. Alternative pathway (C3) activation involves endotoxin.

29 Clonidine:

✗
✗
✓
✓
✗

Clonidine stimulates alpha-2 adrenoceptors to produce analgesia and augment local anaesthetic actions epidurally. It readily enters the CNS but has no respiratory stimulant effects.

30 Xenon:

✓
✓
✓
✗
✓

Xenon is an inert gas which has a blood-gas solubility coefficient of 0.14. It is a potent analgesic comparable to nitrous oxide. It inhibits the NMDA receptor, with little effect on GABA-A or non-NMDA glutamatergic receptors. It has no significant pre-synaptic effects.

31 In determining the pulmonary shunt fraction (Qs/Qt), which of the following information is required:

✗
✓
✗
✓
✓

The shunt equation states that: $Qs/Qt = Cc'O_2 – CaO_2/Cc'O_2 – CvO_2$. P_aCO_2 is needed in the alveolar gas equation which is used to calculate $Cc'O_2$.

32 The recurrent laryngeal nerve innervates the:

✗
✓
✓
✓
✓

The recurrent laryngeal nerve supplies all the intrinsic muscles of the larynx with the exception of the cricothyroid muscle which is supplied by the superior laryngeal nerve. The thyrohyoid, one of the extrinsic laryngeal muscles, is supplied by the hypoglossal nerve.

33 The sacral canal contains:

✗
✗
✓
✗
✗

The dura extends to S2 in the sacral canal which has a volume of approximately 33 ml in the adult. The genitofemoral and ilioinguinal nerves arise from the lumbar plexus.

34 A drug which blocks dopamine receptors only is likely to:

✗
✓
✗
✗
✗

Dopamine receptors exist in splanchnic blood vessels and stimulation causes vasodilatation. Parkinsonism is treated with Levodopa and dopamine antagonists will make it worse.

35 These drugs selectively increase renal blood flow:

✗
✓
✓
✗
✗

Dopamine receptor stimulation results in renal vasodilatation. Dopexamine is an inodilator with dopaminergic activity. Dobutamine acts on beta-1 and beta-2 receptors only.

36 The following factors enhance the diffusion of a drug across the blood brain barrier:

✓
✗
✓
✗
✗

The blood brain barrier comprises tight junctions of capillary endothelium. Lipid solubility facilitates diffusion as does the concentration gradient between plasma and brain.

37 Sevoflurane:

✗
✗
✗
✓
✗

Sevoflurane is a fluorinated ether which boils at 58.6°C and has a blood/gas solubility of 0.69.

38 Intraocular pressure is lowered by:

✓
✓
✗
✓
✓

IOP is influenced by venous drainage, arterial pressure, extraocular muscle tone, and choroidal blood volume which is sensitive to P_aCO_2.

39 **Appropriate nerve blocks for the treatment of pain associated with chronic pancreatitis include:**

✗
✓
✓
✓
✗

Coeliac plexus block is used traditionally to block autonomic afferent activity. Paravertebral block at T8–10 is necessary for pancreatitis. Epidural block of the same segments will abolish the pain of chronic pancreatitis.

40 **Causes of low arterial pressure upon initiation of cardiopulmonary bypass with total crystalloid prime include:**

✓
✗
✗
✗
✗

Arterial pressure is a product of peripheral resistance and cardiac output. Cardiac output is determined by preload, afterload and contractility although, of course, cardiac output is set by the perfusionist during cardiopulminary bypass.

41 **Surgical closure of a patent ductus arteriosus produces:**

✓
✗
✓
✓
✓

An oesophageal stethoscope placed during surgery confirms closure. Resultant decrease in left to right shunting accounts for greater systemic perfusion and decreased venous return from the lungs.

42 **Emergency treatment of severe hypotension unresponsive to ephedrine in a fit patient undergoing cervical laminectomy in the sitting position includes:**

✗
✗
✗
✓
✓

Venous pooling in the seated position renders hypotension likely. Intra-aortic balloon pumping is inappropriate as an immediate treatment. Nitrous oxide (if employed) will increase the volume of an air embolus which is a likely cause of severe hypotension. Sodium bicarbonate will worsen tissue acidosis.

43 **Paraplegic patients with spinal cord transection at T6 for more than one year manifest:**

✓
✓
✓
✗
✗

Autonomic denervation of the sympathetic outflow below T6 predisposes to autonomic hyperreflexia. Intracellular potassium efflux is maximal at 14 days post injury, declines after six months, but may still be present thereafter.

44 For laryngoscopy:

✗ ✗ ✓ ✓ ✗

Atlanto-occipital extension and cervical flexion result in the optimum position. Anterior neck surgery may result in fibrosis. The polio blade angle is 150º.

45 Complications of deep cervical plexus block include:

✗ ✓ ✓ ✓ ✗

The phrenic nerve may be affected, and a Horner's syndrome with ipsilateral meiosis may occur as a result of sympathetic block. Local anaesthetic may diffuse to the recurrent laryngeal nerve leading to hoarseness, and subarachnoid injection is possible.

46 Inadvertent surgical stimulation of the fifth cranial nerve during posterior fossa craniotomy will produce:

✓ ✗ ✗ ✗ ✗

The trigeminal nerve is motor to muscles of mastication and mylohyoid. Stimulation of VIII nerve causes nystagmus. Stimulation of the trigeminal nerve increases circulating catecholamines and causes tachycardia and hypertension.

47 The hypertensive response to laryngoscopy and tracheal intubation may be attenuated by:

✓ ✓ ✗ ✗ ✓

The afferent reflex is depressed by anaesthetic and analgesic agents, and the efferent beta sympathetic effects are attenuated by antagonists. Glycopyrrolate will reduce parasympathetic tone and increase the hypertensive response. Spraying the cords requires laryngoscopy and therefore will cause a hypertensive response.

48 Appropriate recommendations for the peri-operative management of an Afro-Caribbean child scheduled for urgent internal fixation of a closed tibial fracture, whose haemoglobin is found to be 7.5 g dl^{-1} despite minimal blood loss, include:

✓ ✗ ✗ ✗ ✗

Homozygous sickle cell disease can cause anaemia and jaundice. Electrophoresis determines the extent of the disease and hydration should be ensured pending surgery. Hydrocortisone will have no effect and hypotension may precipitate a sickle cell crisis. Succinylcholine can be used safely.

49 **Appropriate management of a female patient with untreated thyrotoxicosis requiring repair of an incarcerated femoral hernia includes:**

✓ ✗ ✗ ✗ ✗

Control of end organ sympathetic stimulation can be achieved with beta blockade in the acute situation. Potassium iodide may be used in addition. Spinal anaesthesia is inappropriate in this case because of the possible need for small bowel surgery. Atropine will worsen arrhythmias and carbimazole cannot be given intravenously.

50 **In assessing the adequacy of medullary perfusion during posterior fossa surgery, the appearance of the following are useful:**

✗ ✗ ✓ ✓ ✓

Medullary cardiovascular centre activity can be judged by monitored cardiovascular variables. Respiratory activity can be useful only if ventilation is spontaneous but is a more sensitive indicator of brain stem dysfunction than cardiovascular changes. EEG changes and body temperature are not useful in this context.

51 **During general anaesthesia for laparoscopy when the intra-abdominal pressure is 40 mmHg the following parameters would decrease:**

✓ ✗ ✓ ✗ ✗

The pressure in the IVC is exceeded by intra-abdominal pressures in excess of 15 mmHg. Decreased venous return to the heart results in decreased filling pressure and decreased cardiac output. Systemic vascular resistance and heart rate will increase due to increased baroreceptor activity.

52 **A continuous positive pressure breathing system (CPAP) for an adult:**

✗ ✓ ✓ ✗ ✓

CPAP can be applied using a mask delivering a fresh gas flow near to the peak inspiratory flow rate. Increasing FRC to greater than closing capacity results in alveolar recruitment and will tend to improve lung compliance.

53 When performing the 'three-in-one' block for pain relief in lower limb surgery:

✗ The femoral nerve lies lateral to the artery. Analgesia will be
✓ obtained over the medial side of the ankle only.
✗
✓
✓

54 The hazard of microshock in hospital can be reduced by use of:

✓ Saline-filled intracardiac catheters can be the cause of microshock.
✗ Multiple earth pads can allow stray currents to develop. Large area
✓ diathermy plates reduce the risk of burns but do not affect the
✗ likelihood of microshock.
✗

55 Malignant hyperthermia:

✓ Malignant hyperpyrexia is inherited as an autosomal dominant
✓ characteristic. There is no sex difference in incidence.
✗
✗
✓

56 A neurolytic coeliac plexus block:

✓ Coeliac plexus block is performed anterolateral to the body of L1
✗ and with the needle posterior to the aorta.
✓
✓
✗

57 Surgical correction of scoliosis:

✗ Spinal cord damage is very rarely associated with surgical
✓ correction of scoliosis. If post-operative ventilation is required
✓ it is usually short-lived.
✓
✗

58 After successful supraclavicular brachial plexus block, sensory anaesthesia will usually be incomplete on the:

✗
✗
✓
✓
✗

Sensory anaesthesia is usually complete on the back of the elbow and the medial and lateral aspects of the forearm. An area on the tip of the shoulder and the medial aspect of the upper arm, supplied by the intercostohumeral nerve, are not blocked.

59 Retro-bulbar block:

✓
✗
✓
✗
✗

Retro-bulbar block tends to cause exophthalmos. It has no effect on lachrymation and because it reduces intraocular pressure will tend to reduce the likelihood of vitreous prolapse.

60 Premature neonates:

✓
✓
✗
✓
✗

Insensible water loss tends to be increased. Neonates have disproportionately fewer Type 1 slow muscle fibres in the diaphragm than children aged two years and are therefore prone to respiratory fatigue.

61 The TURP syndrome:

✓
✓
✗
✗
✓

The TURP syndrome is caused by absorption of irrigating fluid into the circulation. This causes hypokalaemia and hyponatraemia. It is just as likely to occur during spinal anaesthesia as during general anaesthesia.

62 The group A antigen:

✓
✗
✓
✓
✓

The group A antigen is carried on the red blood cells of group A patients and can occur in the saliva of these patients. The most common cause of haemolytic disease of the newborn is Rhesus incompatibility.

63 The penicillins:

✗
✓
✗
✗
✗

The penicillins interfere with bacterial cell wall synthesis, are more effective against organisms which are dividing and are bactericidal. They are effective against some Gram-positive cocci and some are penicillinase resistant.

64 The following are competitive antagonists:

✗
✓
✗
✓
✗

Naltrexone and flumazenil are competitive antagonists. Neostigmine antagonises neuromuscular blockade by preventing the breakdown of acetylcholine. Buprenorphine is a mixed opioid agonist/antagonist. Enoximone is a phosphodiesterase inhibitor preventing the breakdown of cyclic AMP.

65 Intra-operative signs of a haemolytic transfusion reaction include:

✓
✗
✓
✓
✓

Haemolytic transfusion reactions will be associated with an increase in capillary bleeding and hypotension, not hypertension, intra-operatively. Fever, urticaria and periorbital oedema are also intra-operative signs of a severe transfusion reaction.

66 Dopamine:

✗
✓
✓
✗
✓

There is no evidence that dopamine has a renal protective effect or increases creatinine clearance. Dopamine usually increases cardiac output at 2 μg kg^{-1} min^{-1}, increases intracellular calcium concentration and increases splanchnic oxygen requirement.

67 Lactic acid is:

✓
✓
✗
✓
✓

Lactic acid is formed during anaerobic ATP re-synthesis and increases in concentration in the blood during energy deficit. It is formed by red blood cells, converted to glucose by the Cori cycle and oxidised without conversion back to glucose.

68 Low molecular weight heparin:

✗
✓
✗
✗
✓

Low molecular weight heparin (LMWH) does not have any direct inhibitory action on thrombin so its activity is not effectively measured by APTT. It has a longer plasma half-life than standard heparin and has prolonged plasma clearance in renal failure. It is only weakly protein bound and has a high bioavailability. It is only partially reversible by protamine.

69 The blood brain barrier:

✓
✓
✓
✗
✗

The blood brain barrier (BBB) is formed by the tight junctions between endothelial cells and restricts passive diffusion of substrates like glucose which are actively transported through cells into the CNS. CNS infection will impair the function of the BBB. The BBB is more permeable in neonates than adults. Lipophilic drugs readily cross the BBB.

70 In normal individuals with a normal P_aCO_2, cerebral blood flow:

✓
✓
✗
✗
✓

The autoregulatory limits for CBF are cerebral perfusion pressures of 50–140 mmHg so CBF will autoregulate between 50 and 100 mmHg. 100% oxygen causes cerebral vasoconstriction. Hypothermia reduces CBF which has a normal value of 50 ml $100g^{-1}$ min^{-1}. Mannitol reduces blood viscosity and initially increases CBF which will return to normal fairly quickly if autoregulation is intact.

71 In normal pregnancy:

✗
✗
✓
✓
✓

Plasma volume increases to approximately 60 ml kg^{-1} in pregnancy so the total quantity of plasma proteins will increase despite a reduction in plasma concentrations. Bupivacaine is bound to albumin which is reduced in concentration in pregnancy so free plasma levels of bupivacaine are increased.

72 The alpha-2 adrenoreceptor agonist clonidine:

✓
✗
✓
✗
✓

Alpha-2 agonists reduce MAC for inhalational anaesthetics and potentiate the analgesic affects of opioids. They reduce heart rate and arterial pressure. They increase the duration of epidural block with bupivacaine.

73 Intercostal nerves:

✓ The intercostal nerves pass anteriorly to the posterior intercostal
✗ membrane then between the internal intercostals and the innermost
✗ intercostal muscles running inferior to the intercostal vein and
✓ artery. They divide into lateral and anterior cutaneous branches.
✓ Intercostal nerves supply the periphery of the diaphragm.

74 Pulmonary vascular resistance is:

✓ A high haematocrit increases the viscosity of the blood and resistance
✗ to flow. Helium has no effect on pulmonary vascular resistance and
✓ sevoflurane decreases it. Moderate exercise causes pulmonary
✗ vasodilation. PEEP squeezes the pulmonary capillaries and
✓ increases pulmonary vascular resistance.

75 The following are nephrotoxic:

✓ Halothane, unlike the other commonly used volatile anaesthetics, is
✓ not normally metabolised to fluoride. Therefore, nephrotoxic levels
✗ of fluoride are not achieved. All the other agents are nephrotoxic.
✓
✓

76 Shock due to Gram-negative bacteraemia is frequently associated with:

✓ Gram-negative bacteraemia frequently complicates obstructive
✓ jaundice. The shock associated with Gram-negative bacteraemia is
✓ characterised by a high cardiac output with very low systemic
✓ vascular resistance.
✗

77 After a severe burn (greater than 40% full thickness):

✓ Enteral nutrition should be started as soon as possible. Antibiotics
✗ should only be given when there is proven infection to avoid the
✓ development of bacterial resistance.
✓
✗

78 In the critically ill, skeletal muscle:

✓ Early nutritional support does not prevent muscle breakdown.
✓ Endogenous cortisol tends to increase muscle breakdown.
✗
✗
✓

79 The use of propofol for sedation on the Intensive Care Unit is associated with:

✗ The calorie load is approximately 1 kcal ml^{-1} for 1% propofol
✓ solution. Propofol reduces cerebral blood flow and does not
✗ reduce the shunt fraction. It may increase the shunt fraction
✓ due to hypotension.
✗

80 Mixed venous oxygen saturation is:

✗ Mixed venous oxygen saturation is reduced in anaemia because of
✓ the reduced oxygen carrying capacity. It is increased in established systemic
✓ sepsis because of impairment of oxygen utilisation in the tissues with
✗ reduced peripheral extraction of oxygen. Measurement may be intermittent
✓ or by means of a central venous oximetric catheter.

81 The crush syndrome:

✓ Alkalinisation of the urine reduces precipitation of myoglobin in the
✓ renal tubules and ameliorates haem-induced toxicity.
✓
✓
✓

82 Important measures to prevent hospital acquired infections in intensive care include:

✓ Plastic overshoes and routine cultures do not reduce the risk of
✓ infection. Changing the ventilator tubing every 24 hours does not
✗ reduce the risk of developing a chest infection. Sterilisation of
✗ ventilator patient circuits between patients is appropriate.
✗

83 Potential complications of the use of neuromuscular blocking agents in the critically ill include:

✓
✗
✓
✓
✓

Venous thromboembolism is likely if muscle tone in the lower limbs is reduced. Cardiac arrhythmias can be induced by suxamethonium due to changes in serum potassium levels. Protracted muscle weakness and peripheral nerve injury are associated with the use of muscle relaxants. Critical illness neuropathy is not caused by the use of muscle relaxants.

84 Electrocardiographic changes during hypothermia to 28°C include:

✓
✗
✓
✓
✓

Peaked T waves are associated with hyperkalaemia and will tend to be reduced in size during hypothermia. J waves are associated with hypothermia.

85 Ionised calcium:

✓
✓
✓
✓
✗

Normally the blood sample should be allowed to clot and not be anticoagulated but it is possible to measure ionised calcium in a heparinised sample when measuring blood gases. Calcium is bound by the citrate used as an anticoagulant in stored blood. Serum proteins do not affect ionised calcium levels.

86 In thermal dilution techniques for the measurement of cardiac output:

✗
✗
✗
✓
✗

The volume of the injectate is not critical but must be measured accurately. The wedge pressure is not required in the calculation and the patient's temperature has no effect on the measurement. The phase of the respiratory cycle can affect the measurement by as much as 20%.

87 A typical daily regimen for total parenteral nutrition in an adult:

✓
✗
✓
✓
✓

Fat emulsions are not contraindicated in patients with liver failure, but fat clearance from the plasma should be ensured.

88 The effectiveness of defibrillation is increased by:

✗
✗
✗
✓
✓

Delivery during expiration results in a greater conductivity. Large plate contact area with plates correctly applied results in more uniform current spread within the heart and thus improved effectiveness.

89 Signs of overdose of a tricyclic antidepressant include:

✓
✗
✓
✓
✓

Tricyclic antidepressants have a range of actions and the predominant autonomic nervous system effect is anticholinergic. Pupil dilatation rather than constriction would be usual here.

90 In the following situations the measured pulmonary artery occlusion pressure (PAOP) will not reflect left ventricular end-diastolic pressure (LVEDP):

✗
✓
✗
✓
✗

Changes in right-sided pressures as a result of valve disease do not affect per se left-sided pressures. The presence of aortic stenosis does not alter left atrial and hence pulmonary artery occlusion pressure.

91 Hypophosphataemia gives rise to:

✓
✗
✓
✓
✗

Hypophosphataemia shifts the dissociation curve to the left and does not cause a peripheral neuropathy. Muscle weakness is often described in patients with prolonged hypophosphataemia.

92 The following are endogenous pro-inflammatory cytokines:

✓
✓
✗
✗
✗

Interleukin 10 and interleukin 1 receptor antagonist act as anti-inflammatory cytokines. Nuclear factor kappa B is a transcription factor which promotes the formation of a range of proteins including cytokines but it is not itself a cytokine.

93 The treatment of amitriptyline poisoning includes:

✗ ✗ ✗ ✗ ✓

Forced diuresis does not speed elimination significantly. Isoprenaline will increase the risk of tachyarrhythmias as will atropine. Amitriptyline has anticholinergic properties. Digitalis may increase the risk of arrhythmias. Beta adrenoceptor antagonists are appropriate for the treatment of tachyarrhythmias.

94 Conditions associated with smoke inhalation injury include:

✗ ✓ ✓ ✗ ✓

Heat causes sloughing and oedema of the mucosa of the upper airway. Smoke inhalation is often associated with carbon monoxide (the presence of carboxyhaemoglobin shifts the oxyhaemoglobin dissociation curve to the left) and cyanide inhalation.

95 Nosocomial pneumonia is:

✗ ✓ ✓ ✓ ✓

Urinary tract infection is the most common hospital acquired infection. H2 antagonists increase the incidence of gastric colonisation and hence nosocomial pneumonia in ventilated patients. Effective hand washing has been shown to be the best precaution used in the prevention of nosocomial pneumonia.

96 Likely causes of severe hypotension following surgical removal of a phaeochromocytoma include:

✗ ✗ ✗ ✓ ✓

Patients are prepared for surgery using catecholamine antagonists and should not therefore be vasoconstricted. Adrenal cortical failure would result in mild hypotension over a more chronic time frame. Plasma volume is diminished in such patients even with pre-operative preparation and along with splanchnic pooling are the most likely causes of hypotension in such a patient.

97 Criteria applied in the diagnosis of 'brain death' include:

✓ ✓ ✗ ✗ ✗

The diagnosis of brain death is dependent upon demonstrating lack of activity in the medulla and brain stem. Up-going plantars are a spinal response. EEG evidence is not required for the diagnosis of brain stem death.

98 The effects of Ecstasy (3,4-methylenedioxymethamphetamine):

✗
✓
✗
✗
✓

Ecstasy increases monoamine release from nerve terminals and also reduces the reuptake of serotonin. It has similar but weaker effects on dopamine. The toxic effects, such as hyperpyrexia, are often not dose related. Thirst occurs from ADH release and loss of salt during excess sweating; increased water intake may lead to hyponatraemia.

99 Endotoxin:

✗
✗
✓
✗
✗

The limulus lysate (from the horseshoe crab) assay is a method of measuring endotoxin concentrations. Endotoxin is detected in approximately half of those patients with Gram-negative bacteraemia although this varies with the type of organism. Endotoxin has three main components and can be degraded by antibodies against the lipid A component.

100 In acute hepatic failure:

✓
✓
✗
✗
✗

Assuming the liver is not totally destroyed, protein production is often increased. Alkaline phosphatase, lactate dehydrogenase and bilirubin are not sensitive indicators of liver damage.

101 In children, death from severe burns in the second week after injury is often due to:

✗
✗
✗
✗
✓

Haemoconcentration, anaemia and protein destruction are all acute events and should not be associated with late death. Death from liver failure within two weeks of burn injury would be most unlikely.

102 The risk of infection in a central venous catheter:

✓
✗
✓
✗
✗

Some micro-organisms adhere better to polyvinylchloride than to Teflon catheters. In the ICU patient catheters tend to move more when placed in the internal jugular vein thus more readily allowing the entry of bacteria. The cut down technique is often performed under suboptimal antiseptic conditions. Occlusive dressings allow the accumulation of a medium ideal for the growth of bacteria.

103 A rapid shallow breathing pattern in the critically ill:

✓ The cause of rapid shallow breathing in the critically ill is unknown
✓ although stretch receptor stimulation may be involved. It is a
✗ common cause of failure to wean from ventilation.
✗
✓

104 Fluoroquinolones:

✓ The spectrum of activity varies within the class of fluoroquinolones
✓ but all are active against Gram-positive as well as Gram-negative
✓ bacteria. Many antibiotics when given orally are chelated by
✓ aluminium salts and are then not absorbed.
✓

105 The following measurements are consistent with physiological oliguria:

✓ Physiological oliguria results in concentrated urine with sodium
✓ retention. The normal urinary creatinine concentration is around
✓ 10 mmol L^{-1} while that of plasma is around 60 µmol L^{-1}.
✓
✗

106 Side effects of amiodarone include:

✓ Although widely used, amiodarone causes a range of side effects
✓ some of which are frequent and serious, although some reverse on
✓ stopping the drug, others are permanent.
✓
✗

107 Patients at greater than normal risk of developing Gram-negative bacteraemia include those suffering from:

✓ This is a commonly seen problem in the ICU. Polycythaemia is a
✓ red cell condition and immune function is normal. Infection is a
✓ common feature of diabetes mellitus.
✗
✓

108 In a patient suffering from paroxysmal nocturnal dyspnoea the following signs would favour asthma rather than left ventricular failure:

✗
✗
✓
✓
✗

Expiratory wheeze is a sign of bronchospasm. Central cyanosis occurs later in left ventricular failure. A raised JVP, basal crepitations and hypotension are features of cardiac failure.

109 Trans-oesophageal echocardiography:

✗
✓
✓
✓
✓

Echocardiography cannot quantify intracardiac pressures but can image flow. It can help assess myocardial ischaemia and contractility by imaging motion of the walls of the heart. Ejection fraction can be estimated using the echocardiogram.

110 Morbid obesity:

✓
✗
✗
✓
✓

The blood volume is higher in morbidly obese patients but on a weight per volume basis is lower; 50 versus 70 ml kg^{-1}. Oxygen flux is increased in obesity. Hypoxic pulmonary vasoconstriction is unaffected. Left ventricular hypertrophy is common because of the associated hypertension, and insulin resistance is associated with obesity.

111 In an otherwise normal person, chronic iron deficiency anaemia with a haemoglobin concentration of 60 g L^{-1} is associated with:

✗
✓
✗
✓
✗

The mixed venous PO_2 is reduced because less oxygen is available for delivery to metabolically active tissues. Heart rate increases to increase cardiac output to compensate for the reduced oxygen carriage. Metabolic acidosis does not occur because of compensatory mechanisms to maintain oxygen delivery. The left atrial PO_2 will be normal but the oxygen content will be reduced. The oxyhaemoglobin dissociation curve is shifted to the right to enable more oxygen to be off-loaded to the tissues.

112 **The pulmonary artery wedge pressure is a good indicator of left ventricular end-diastolic pressure in patients suffering from:**

✓
✗
✓
✓
✓

In mitral stenosis the left atrial pressure is greater than the LVEDP because of the resistance to flow through the valve.

113 **The development of high titres of anti D antibodies in a Rhesus negative mother with an Rh positive fetus:**

✓
✓
✓
✗
✗

Haemolysis in the fetus causes anaemia and jaundice. The antigen is on the red cells and cannot enter the maternal circulation independently. The development of high titres usually occurs later in pregnancy.

114 **An acutely developing blood coagulation defect associated with massive transfusion may be due to:**

✓
✓
✓
✓
✓

Thrombocytopenia and deficiency of Factors V and VIII occur by dilution during massive transfusion. DIC and fibrinolysis can be precipitated by major haemorrhage and massive transfusion. Incompatible blood transfusion will cause a coagulopathy.

115 **Platelet concentrate:**

✗
✗
✓
✓
✗

Platelet concentrate has a maximum shelf-life of five days and platelet function is best maintained at 22°C. Citrate is used as an anticoagulant. Cross-matching is required because of antibodies in serum. Plasma histamine levels do not change significantly on administration.

116 **In pulmonary contusion there will be:**

✓
✓
✓
✓
✗

Lung compliance is reduced with pulmonary contusion.

117 Recognised complications of bronchial neoplasms include:

✓ Bronchial neoplasms can secrete calcitonin, ADH and ACTH.
✗ They do not cause hyperkalaemia or hypothyroidism.
✓
✓
✗

118 The following symptoms strongly suggest a diagnosis of transient cerebral ischaemia:

✓ The predominant feature of transient ischaemic attacks is one of
✗ fleeting focal neurological dysfunction lasting minutes or hours.
✗ This would therefore rule out B, C and D.
✗
✓

119 A history of alcoholism is associated with:

✓
✗
✓
✓
✗

Alcoholics tend to be overweight but malnourished because alcohol is a good source of calories but alcoholics tend otherwise not to eat well. They therefore have reduced plasma albumin concentrations. Usually, a mild macrocytic anaemia is seen possibly due to direct effects of alcohol on the bone marrow rather than a vitamin deficiency. Alcoholics are at risk of hypotension due to a polyneuropathy causing impaired vasoconstrictor reflexes.

120 Effects of hypermagnesaemia include:

✓
✓
✗
✗
✓

Magnesium is the second most abundant cation of the intracellular space after potassium. Magnesium acts as a non-competitive inhibitor of the IP3-gated calcium channel and of IP3 binding – therefore it may be considered as an intracellular calcium antagonist. High magnesium concentrations inhibit the release of acetylcholine from the presynaptic nerve terminal and also have an inhibitory effect on the postjunctional potentials. It was thought that high magnesium concentrations potentiated the effect of depolarising muscle relaxants. However, a recent study has shown an antagonism of the block caused by suxamethonium. Hypermagnesaemia is associated with a shortened onset time and a reduced ED50 for most non-depolarising muscle relaxants. Magnesium is used as an anti-arrhythmic agent and decreases myocardial excitability and contractility.

121 Bilateral hilar lymphadenopathy is a feature of:

✓
✓
✗
✗
✗

The usual diagnosis of bilateral hilar lymphadenopathy is sarcoid but included in the differential diagnosis is lymphoma (both Hodgkin's and non-Hodgkin's) and tuberculosis (although here unilateral lymphadenopathy may be more usual).

122 A low fixed cardiac output is associated with:

✓
✓
✓
✗
✗

Cor pulmonale may be associated with a low cardiac output but it is not fixed. Digoxin is an inotrope.

123 Collapse of the lower lobe of the right lung is characterised by:

✓
✗
✗
✗
✓

Collapse of a lobe of a lung causes hypoxia and induces tachypnoea resulting in a decreased P_aCO_2. Stony dullness to percussion is seen in consolidation rather than collapse.

124 A haemoglobin of 80 g L^{-1} with a reticulocyte count of 10% is associated with:

✗
✗
✗
✓
✗

Anaemia in the presence of a high reticulocyte count is seen in haemolysis and suggests active red cell regeneration in the presence of red cell loss. Aplastic anaemia, untreated pernicious anaemia, polycythaemia and acute leukaemia are not associated with a high reticulocyte count.

125 Causes of atrial fibrillation include:

✓
✓
✓
✗
✗

A, B and C are true. Rheumatic heart disease and thyrotoxicosis commonly cause atrial fibrillation. Atropine increases heart rate and may result in a sinus tachycardia but not atrial fibrillation.

126 There is a recognised association between ulcerative colitis and:

✓ Like many other conditions listed here, ulcerative colitis is a bowel
✓ manifestation of what may be a more generalised inflammatory
✓ state. The true cause of clubbing is still unknown.
✓
✓

127 Endocrine syndromes associated with primary bronchogenic carcinoma include:

✓ Bronchogenic tumours are known to secrete ADH, PTH and serotonin
✗ with biochemical effects that may require treatment prior to anaesthesia
✓ and surgery. Normoglycaemia or rarely hypoglycaemia would be more likely.
✓
✓

128 Pleural effusion is a common complication of:

✗ Although some of the other organisms may be associated with an
✗ empyema, only pneumococcal pneumonia is commonly associated
✗ with a simple pleural effusion.
✓
✗

129 In primary adrenocortical failure:

✓ Primary adrenocortical insufficiency, Addison's disease, results in
✗ decreased release of glucocorticoids and mineralocorticoids. Blood
✗ cortisol, sodium and glucose concentrations are low, whilst
✓ potassium and ACTH are high. A normal response to exogenous
✓ ACTH excludes the diagnosis of primary adrenocortical failure.

130 You would expect to find sensory changes in the following conditions:

✓ Poliomyelitis and motor neurone disease affect motor not sensory
✗ nerves. Carpal tunnel syndrome affects the entire nerve – both
✓ motor and sensory fibres.
✗
✓

131 The metabolic response to major surgery includes:

✗
✓
✗
✓
✓

The stress response includes increased release of catecholamines, glucocorticoids and ADH. There is therefore water and sodium retention and blood glucose rises due to the anti-insulin effects of the steroids and catecholamines.

132 In a patient with renal failure, if given repeatedly, the following drugs or their active metabolites are more likely to accumulate than in a normal person:

✓
✓
✗
✗
✗

The excretion of morphine metabolites is dependent on renal function. The terminal half-life of vecuronium is increased by approximately 1.5 by renal failure and it is cumulative after repeated doses. Thiopental is less protein bound in renal failure requiring a reduced dose to provide a given effect but is no more likely to accumulate in renal failure.

133 Hepatitis B infection:

✗
✓
✓
✓
✓

Immunisation against Hepatitis B is mandatory and requires booster injections every five years. Transmission occurs via blood, seminal and vaginal secretions. Cirrhosis, chronic active hepatitis or liver carcinoma may supervene.

134 Radiological evidence of enlargement of the pulmonary artery is a recognised feature of:

✓
✓
✓
✗
✓

Hyperdynamic right ventricular output resulting from left-right shunting leads to pulmonary hypertension and arterial enlargement. Pulmonary valve stenosis occurs in Fallot's tetralogy.

135 The following are recognised causes of thrombocytopenia:

✓
✓
✓
✓
✗

SLE leads to thrombocytopenia in 10% of cases. Hypersplenism in cirrhosis and infectious mononucleosis may cause thrombocytopenia in contrast to the situation after splenectomy.

136 The carcinoid syndrome is associated with elevated plasma levels of:

✗
✗
✗
✗
✓

Argentaffin cells in carcinoid tumours secrete vasoactive amines including histamine, bradykinin and serotonin. Hepatic secondaries result in carcinoid syndrome.

137 Clinical findings consistent with persistent vomiting for two months include:

✓
✓
✓
✓
✓

Persistent loss of gastric secretions leads to dehydration and hypochloraemic alkalosis. Alkalosis can result in tetany and hypokalaemia. Lack of intrinsic factor in gastric secretions contributes to pernicious anaemia.

138 Ankylosing spondylitis:

✗
✓
✓
✓
✓

The male:female ratio is about 4:1. Iritis occurs in up to 25% of cases. There is a predilection for the sacroiliac joints as well as the spine.

139 The following may relieve severe pain from osseous metastases of carcinoma of the prostate:

✓
✗
✓
✗
✓

Androgen deprivation, achieved by orchidectomy or radiotherapy, is useful for local spread or metastatic spread. Stilboestrol is a useful palliative.

140 Subarachnoid haemorrhage:

✓
✓
✓
✗
✗

Commonly occurs from rupture of a congenital aneurysm, possibly precipitated by physical strain, and causes a sudden large increase in ICP. It is twice as common in females as in males. Dehydration does not cause subarachnoid haemorrhage.

141 **Patients with acromegaly have a:**

✗ Decreased sensitivity to insulin – diabetes mellitus is not uncommon.
✗ Overproduction of growth hormone is from an eosinophilic adenoma.
✓
✗
✓

142 **The following are true of osmosis:**

✗ Osmolarity refers to the number of osmoles per litre of specific
✗ solvent. Osmolality refers to the number of osmoles per kg of
✗ specific solvent. The depression of the freezing point of a solution is
✓ directly proportional to its osmolality.
✓

143 **In a time-cycled ventilator providing constant pressure generation during the inspiratory phase:**

✗ A source driving gas at 4 bar is not essential. The tidal volume will
✓ be determined by the pressure set on the ventilator and the lung
✓ compliance. The peak inspiratory pressure is set on the ventilator
✗ and does not give an indication of airways resistance.
✗

144 **Applications of the Doppler effect in clinical practice involve measurement of a change in:**

✗ The Doppler effect refers to ultrasonic waves not to electrical
✗ conductivity, frequency response of the arterial wall, temperature
✓ or harmonic waves.
✗
✗

145 **Gas properties that influence resistance during laminar flow include:**

✗ Resistance during laminar flow depends on viscosity. Critical
✓ temperature, density, diffusion rate and molecular weight have
✗ no effect.
✗
✗

146 FEV$_1$/FVC ratio measurement is useful in the detection of:

✗
✗
✓
✗
✗

Restrictive pulmonary lesions are detected from measurements of vital capacity. More complicated tests are required to measure functional residual capacity and elastic recoil of the lung. The FEV$_1$/FVC ratio is a measurement made on expiration.

147 Potential complications of radial artery cannulation for continuous measurement of arterial blood pressure include:

✓
✗
✓
✗
✓

Cerebral arterial emboli are caused by internal carotid or vertebral artery cannulation. Sensation of the thenar eminence is supplied by the median nerve. Pulmonary oedema is not associated with radial artery cannulation.

148 In cardiac output measurement by thermodilution:

✗
✗
✓
✗
✓

The thermistor is accurate to 0.1°C. Measurements are still accurate after 48 hours in situ. Measurements will tend to over read during inspiration.

149 Carbon dioxide crosses biological membranes 20 times more readily than oxygen because carbon dioxide:

✗
✓
✗
✗
✗

The Reynolds number and molecular weight are not relevant to diffusion of gases. Carbon dioxide does not have an electric charge and is not actively transported across biological membranes.

150 Calculation of systemic vascular resistance requires measurement of:

✗
✗
✓
✓
✗

Systemic vascular resistance is calculated from the mean arterial pressure (some equations deduct the CVP first) divided by cardiac output. Coronary blood flow, pulmonary artery pressure and rate of peripheral arteriolar flow are irrelevant.

151 Helium:

✓
✗
✓
✗
✗

Helium is stored as a gas in cylinders and does not support combustion. It does not affect the work of breathing in bronchospasm because bronchospasm affects the smaller airways where flow is laminar.

152 Vacuum insulated evaporators (VIE) containing liquid oxygen:

✗
✓
✓
✗
✓

Oxygen is stored below its critical temperature of -119°C not -183°C. The oxygen is cooled when some is drawn off due to latent heat of vaporisation.

153 The pneumotachograph:

✓
✓
✓
✓
✗

The pneumotachograph works by measuring pressure change across a resistance with laminar flow. It has a response time sufficiently rapid for breath-by-breath monitoring. Changes in gas composition will alter viscosity and may affect accuracy as can temperature changes.

154 Intra-operative heat loss due to convection may be minimised by:

✓
✗
✗
✗
✗

Increasing theatre humidity or humidifying inspired gases does not affect convection losses, only evaporation losses. Heated mattresses do not prevent convection losses from exposed body cavities. Evaporation of spirit from the skin is another form of evaporative heat loss.

155 When the statistical P value is reported as being < 0.001:

✓
✗
✓
✗
✗

By convention any P value of less than 0.05 indicates rejection of the null hypothesis and that the difference between two sample means is statistically significant. This does not mean that the results are definitely clinically significant. The P value does not describe the distribution of the data.

156 In a circle breathing system:

✗
✗
✓
✓
✓

Two uni-directional valves are required for efficient function. The intergranular space in a soda lime canister should approximate to a normal tidal volume.

157 Measurement of peak expiratory flow rate:

✓ ✗ ✗ ✗ ✓

Peak expiratory flow rate can be calculated from the Vitalograph but is not as accurate as the Wright peak flow meter. The Wright peak flow meter uses the principle of a variable orifice with a constant pressure drop. Peak expiratory flow rate cannot be measured using a capnograph.

158 Oxygen concentrators:

✓ ✓ ✗ ✓ ✗

Oxygen concentrators can be used on aircraft. They must deliver a concentration of argon higher than air because they work by 'concentrating' atmospheric air by absorbing nitrogen in zeolite. Argon is not removed so its concentration in the remaining gas will increase.

159 The air in an operating theatre:

✗ ✗ ✓ ✗ ✗

The dew point must be at or below room temperature. Infrared analysers are not sufficiently sensitive to detect volatile agent concentrations in parts per million. Room air is one of the calibration points for oxygen analysers. The minimum number of air changes per hour is 20.

160 The end-tidal partial pressure of carbon dioxide:

✓ ✓ ✗ ✗ ✗

Nitrous oxide absorbs infrared radiation and will increase the reading on a capnograph if an inappropriate wavelength is used. It has the same molecular weight as carbon dioxide and can lead to an overestimate of the measurement of carbon dioxide by mass spectrometry. Water vapour does not reduce the mass spectrometer reading for carbon dioxide. PEEP does not influence measurement of end-tidal carbon dioxide tension. End-tidal carbon dioxide tension can never exceed the P_aCO_2.

161 On the day of major abdominal surgery, a normal adult will have:

✗ ✗ ✗ ✓ ✗

1.5 litres of 5% dextrose only provides 300 kcal whereas the normal calorie requirement (depending on sex and size) will be approximately 2000–3000 kcal. Daily potassium requirements are in the range of 1–2 mmol kg^{-1}. Two litres of Hartmann's only contains about 10 mmol K^+. Maximum concentrating ability of normal adult kidneys is up to 1200 mOsm L^{-1}. Maintenance fluid requirements in the adult are about 2 ml kg^{-1} h^{-1}.

162 Likely findings in an elderly dehydrated patient with prolonged intestinal obstruction who is hypotensive, tachypnoeic and confused, breathing air include:

✓ Hypomagnesaemia is associated with gastrointestinal disease due to
✓ excess loss via gut secretions and associated NG drainage. Shocked
✓ patients usually have increased levels of insulin antagonists such as
✓ glucagon, cortisol and adrenaline. This results in hyperglycaemia.
✓ A high urea is a common accompaniment of dehydration.

163 Pre-operative preparation of a patient with primary hyperparathyroidism will necessitate the use of:

✓ Primary hyperparathyroidism results in hypercalcaemia which antagonises
✓ ADH and results in sodium and water loss. Giving 0.9% sodium chloride
✗ will replace this loss, dilute Ca^{++} and also increase urine flow and Ca^{++}
✗ excretion. It is recommended that urine output be maintained at
✗ 200–300 ml h^{-1} in the adult and this is best achieved by judicious use of fluids alongside diuretics such as furosemide.

164 Airway characteristics of an adult with acromegaly include:

✗ Patients with acromegaly actually have decreased airway patency and
✓ hypertrophy of the mucosa of the nasopharynx which are over, not under,
✗ developed. The larynx is frequently narrowed with subglottic stenosis a
✗ common feature leading to difficulty of passage of endotracheal tubes.
✓

165 The success of cricoid pressure in preventing aspiration into the lungs during a rapid sequence induction depends upon:

✓ The use of cricoid pressure in preventing aspiration is dependent upon
✓ adequate compression of the oesophagus against a vertebral body to
✓ prevent passive regurgitation. An incomplete cricoid cartilage or
✓ presence of a nasogastric tube will prevent adequate compression
✗ of the oesophagus. Pre-oxygenation has no effect on preventing aspiration.

166 If the rapid intravenous administration of thiopental and succinylcholine is followed within one minute by the onset of muscle stiffness, the differential diagnosis should include:

✗ Onset of muscle stiffness following succinylcholine is a characteristic
✓ feature of both myotonia congenita and malignant hyperthermia.
✗ Atypical plasma cholinesterase and familial periodic paralysis cause a
✓ decrease in muscle tone. Muscle tone is not increased in motor
✗ neurone disease.

167 Features of pulmonary function after upper abdominal surgery include:

✓
✗
✗
✓
✓

Functional residual capacity is markedly decreased following upper abdominal surgery even with effective pain relief. Respiratory rate is increased and the shift of the majority of ventilation to the apices of the lungs is due to reduced functional residual capacity with a resulting decrease in compliance of the alveoli at the lung base.

168 In induced hypothermia:

✓
✗
✗
✓
✗

Hypothermia decreases anaesthetic requirements. Ventricular fibrillation does not usually occur until core temperature reaches approximately 28°C. There is a paradoxical increase in urine output (cold diuresis) due to decreased renal tubular reabsorptive capacity. Oxygen dissociation curve is shifted to the left in hypothermia.

169 To repair lacerations on the palm of the hand the following nerves must be blocked:

✗
✓
✗
✓
✗

Only the ulnar and medians nerve supply the palm of the hand.

170 Compartment syndrome:

✗
✗
✓
✗
✓

Compartment syndrome can occur in any extremity (both upper and lower) where there are deep fascial compartments. Absence of sensation to light touch, paraesthesia and pain on passive muscle movement are characteristic presenting features. Loss of distal pulses is a very late clinical sign and thus pulses may still be present long after significant tissue and muscle necrosis has occurred.

171 Fat embolism syndrome:

✓
✓
✓
✗
✓

Hypoxaemia often presents before clinical signs of respiratory distress. Petechial rashes are a hallmark of FES and may also be seen in the retina. FES is much more common following long bone fractures (e.g. lower limb). Although isolated cases of cerebral FES are described with focal neurological signs, they are uncommon.

172 Nitric oxide:

✓
✗
✓
✗
✓

Nitric oxide is synthesised from arginine in a reaction catalysed by nitric oxide synthase. Nitric oxide stimulates guanylyl cyclase which increases cGMP, resulting in a fall in intracellular calcium concentration and relaxation of bronchial smooth muscle.

173 Toxic effects of oxygen therapy include:

✗
✓
✓
✗
✗

Convulsions, usually clonic-tonic, are part of the 'Paul Bert effect'. The pulmonary epithelium is damaged by high concentrations of oxygen causing loss of surfactant and interstitial thickening.

174 Intra-abdominal pressure in excess of 25 mmHg (abdominal compartment syndrome):

✓
✓
✗
✓
✓

High intra-abdominal pressure causes lymphoedema by impeding venous and lymphatic return from the lower limbs. Renal failure may result from reduction in renal perfusion pressure (renal arterial pressure –renal venous pressure).

175 The radial nerve:

✓
✗
✓
✗
✓

The deltoid muscle is innervated by the axillary nerve (C5, C6). The radial nerve has important cutaneous branches which supply sensation to most of the dorsum of the hand.

176 In the fetal circulation:

✓
✓
✗
✗
✓

There is one umbilical vein. Approximately 50% of the blood returning to the fetus passes through the fetal liver. The remaining 50% passes through the ductus venosus to the inferior vena cava.

177 Pain in the area of an upper arm tourniquet is mediated via the:

✓
✗
✗
✓
✗

Cutaneous branches of the circumflex nerve innervate the skin overlying the lower part of deltoid muscle. The posteromedial aspect of the upper arm is innervated by the intercostobrachial nerve.

178 Angiotensin converting enzyme inhibitors cause:

✓
✓
✗
✓
✓

ACE inhibitors do not increase total body water.

179 Hepatic blood flow decreases:

✓
✗
✓
✓
✗

Hepatic oxygen extraction is limited by the reduction in hepatic blood flow.

180 The following are true of the use of dibucaine in the detection of abnormal serum cholinesterase:

✓
✓
✗
✓
✓

The dibucaine number is approximately 20 in patients who are homozygous for the atypical enzyme.

MCQ examination Single Best Answer (SBA)

SBA Paper 1

Question 1

A neonate born at 28 weeks gestation and now six weeks old develops apnoeic episodes following an inguinal herniotomy performed under GA.

Which of the following blood results/vital signs are *LEAST* likely to be associated with apnoeic spells in this age group?

a blood glucose 1.7 mmol L^{-1}

b core temperature 35.2°C

c core temperature 39.5°C

d **haemoglobin 11.5 g dl^{-1}**

e serum ionised calcium 0.8 mmol L^{-1}

Hyperthermia, hypothermia, hypoglycaemia and hypocalcaemia are all associated with apnoeic episodes in pre-term infants; although the haemoglobin is below normal for a neonate, at this level it is unlikely to be associated with apnoeas.

Question 2

A 37-year-old man has an uneventful total colectomy performed under GA. Surgery, lasting five hours, was performed in the Lloyd-Davis position. One hour post-operatively, with a 0.1% L-bupivacaine thoracic epidural infusion in progress, he has no abdominal pain but does have pain in both calves. There are decreased lower limb movements bilaterally with reduced pinprick sensation in all dermatomes below the knees.

What is the most appropriate initial investigation in this scenario?

a **compartment pressure measurement in both calves**

b doppler arterial pulse measurement in both legs

c electromyography of leg flexor and extensor muscles

d magnetic resonance imaging of the thoraco-lumbar spine

e ultrasound scan of deep venous system in both calves

Compartment syndrome is a well described complication following prolonged surgery in the Lloyd Davis position; breakthrough pain in the calves despite a functioning epidural is an important clue; the neurological findings do not suggest spinal cord compression so MRI and EMG are not indicated ; bilateral deep vein thromboses are highly unlikely.

Question 3

A previously fit 54-year-old woman presents to the Emergency Department with severe sore throat and increasingly noisy breathing for the past 12 hours. She finds it difficult to swallow her saliva and cannot tolerate lying flat. Her tympanic temperature is 39.2°C, pulse rate 110 beats min^{-1}, BP 130/85, SpO_2 92% on 35% oxygen via facemask. There is marked inspiratory stridor.

What is the most appropriate management plan?

a administer intravenous steroids and antibiotics, nebulised adrenaline and high flow oxygen by CPAP facemask in a high dependency area

b after direct examination of the oropharynx, the patient should have blood cultures taken, receive oral antibiotics, high flow oxygen and be observed in a high dependency area

c the airway should be secured by awake fibreoptic intubation under local anaesthesia, followed by admission to an Intensive Care Unit

d **the airway should be secured by tracheal intubation following direct laryngoscopy under deep inhalational anaesthesia**

e the patient should be transferred, fully monitored, to the operating theatre for immediate tracheostomy under local anaesthesia

The clinical picture is highly suggestive of inflammatory upper airway obstruction, most probably acute epiglottitis; the patient needs to have their airway secured by intubation. Deep inhalational anaesthesia is the safest technique in this scenario. An awake fibreoptic technique may result in acute airway obstruction or laryngeal spasm in this situation.

Question 4

A 7-year-old child weighing 24 kg is having squint correction surgery under general anaesthesia. During the procedure, his heart rate falls abruptly to 45 beats per minute and his blood pressure is 70/40.

What is the most appropriate initial action to take?

a **ask the surgeon to release the globe of the eye**

b give atropine 480 µg intravenously

c give ephedrine 6 mg intravenously

d give glycopyrollate 240 µg intravenously

e reduce the inspired concentration of sevoflurane

Severe bradyarrythmias due to the oculo-cardiac reflex are a potential problem with squint surgery. Releasing traction on the eye is the first action to take followed by a bolus of an anticholinergic agent to obtund the reflex.

Question 5

A 45-year-old woman with a past history of mild asthma and anxiety undergoes left shoulder arthroscopic surgery under interscalene brachial plexus block. Post-operatively she complains of dyspnoea and light-headedness. Breath sounds are slightly reduced on the left side of the chest. SpO_2 92% (on air), BP 110/70, peak flow 290 L min^{-1}. A standard portable CXR appears normal.

What is the most likely cause of her symptoms?

a exacerbation of asthma

b **left phrenic nerve palsy**

c left recurrent laryngeal nerve palsy

d psychogenic dyspnoea

e subarachnoid local anaesthetic injection

The clinical signs and slightly reduced peak flow do not suggest an exacerbation of asthma. Recurrent laryngeal nerve can complicate interscalene blockade but would cause hoarseness rather than dyspnoea. Psychogenic dyspnoea is a possibility but does not account for the low SpO_2. The time scale of symptoms does not fit with subarachnoid injection. Phrenic nerve palsy would account for all her symptoms and signs. NB An inspiratory CXR is required to demonstrate a raised hemidiaphragm with phrenic nerve palsy

Question 6

A 72-year-old man is ventilated on ICU four hours following elective coronary artery surgery. His pulse is 110 beats min^{-1}, BP 85/45, CVP 17 mmHg, urine output 25 ml hr^{-1} in the last two hours and tympanic temperature 37.6°C. Heart sounds are difficult to hear but breath sounds are normal. A 12-lead ECG is unchanged from pre-operatively.

What is the most likely cause of the patient's current clinical condition?

a developing septic shock

b hypovolaemia

c myocardial ischaemia

d **pericardial tamponade**

e tension pneumothorax

In the context of post-operative cardiac surgery, pericardial tamponade is the most likely explanation of the patient's clinical signs and cardiovascular parameters

Question 7

A 56-year-old woman who had a total colectomy develops a tachyarrhythmia 12 hours post-operatively on the HDU. She has a past history of hypertension treated by bendroflumethiazide but no history of cardiac problems.

Which of the following serum electrolyte abnormalities is the most likely to contribute to the arrhythmia?

a ionised calcium 1.88 mmol L^{-1}

b **magnesium 0.38 mmol L^{-1}**

c phosphate 0.58 mmol L^{-1}

d potassium 3.4 mmol L^{-1}

e sodium 129 mmol L^{-1}

The patient has significant hypomagnesaemia, probably due to diuretic therapy, and this is the most likely exacerbating factor for the development of an arrhythmia in this case. The serum potassium is only just below the normal range so unlikely to be the main precipitant.

Question 8

You need to anaesthetise a woman who does not speak English, for a category 3 Caesarean section.

What is the best way to take a history and provide information to this patient?

a **professional telephone translation service**

b the O and G registrar who has some understanding of the patient's language

c the patient's husband who has a limited command of English

d the patient's 11-year-old daughter who is bilingual

e written translated materials

Family members (especially children) or those with a limited command of the languages required should not be used for medical translation purposes other than in an emergency. We do not know if the patient can read or what she understands if she can. Unless a professional translator is available in person then the telephone helpline would be the best option.

Question 9

A 10-month-old apparently well infant presents for religious circumcision under GA. Routine examination reveals a soft systolic murmur; the rest of the examination is normal.

The most appropriate action to take is:

a postpone surgery and obtain an urgent cardiac echo

b **postpone surgery and refer the child back to the GP**

c proceed with anaesthesia because this is an 'innocent' murmur

d proceed with anaesthesia giving antibiotic cover

e proceed with surgery under local anaesthesia

A cardiac murmur in a child below one year cannot be dismissed as innocent without an echocardiogram. The case is not urgent and the child is well so it should be referred back to the GP to organise a cardiology outpatient referral.

Question 10

You administer a general anaesthetic to a previously fit young man for arthroscopic repair of a ruptured left anterior cruciate ligament. The thigh tourniquet was inflated to 200 mmHg above the systolic blood pressure for 110 minutes. Post-operatively, he complains of paraesthesiae in his left calf and sole of the foot.

Which of the following is the single most likely cause of the paraesthesiae?

a compartment syndrome in the thigh

b **compression injury to the sciatic nerve**

c deep venous thrombosis in the calf

d ischaemic injury to the calf muscles

e pressure injury from the edge of the operating table

DVT is unlikely, as is calf muscle ischaemia or compartment syndrome after less than two hours tourniquet time. Paraesthesia in the sciatic nerve distribution is more likely to be due to tourniquet compression than neuropraxia from the operating table.

Question 11

A 40-year-old man is scheduled for elective knee arthroscopy. You commence intravenous induction with thiopental but after injecting 100 mg the patient complains of an intense burning pain in his hand associated with blanching of the fingers.

What is the most important next step to take in managing this situation?

a arrange for a stellate ganglion block to be performed in the affected limb

b insert an IV cannula in the contralateral limb and administer opioid analgesia

c insert an IV cannula in the contralateral limb and administer papaverine

d **leave the IV cannula *in situ* and flush with heparinised saline**

e remove the IV cannula, apply local pressure and elevate the limb

The history is highly suggestive of intra-arterial injection of thiopental. The priority is to dilute the irritant by flushing the vessel with isotonic or heparinised saline.

Question 12

A 75-year-old man is scheduled for a total knee replacement under general anaesthesia supplemented by a femoral nerve block for peri-operative analgesia.

What is the most effective way to reduce the likelihood of local anaesthetic toxicity during placement of the block?

a adding a vasoconstrictor to the local anaesthetic

b **injecting the local anaesthetic slowly and aspirating at regular intervals**

c monitoring the patient with ECG, SpO_2 and non-invasive blood pressure

d not exceeding the maximum permissible dose of local anaesthetic

e using a nerve stimulator to guide block placement

B is the correct answer because it is the only option that allows inadvertent intravascular injection to be detected. A and D are more related to toxicity due to absorption which would occur later. C is about detecting effects of toxicity. E could allow use of lower doses of LA and theoretically should make intravascular injection less likely but is not as reliable as B.

Question 13

A 60-year-old man is scheduled for a palmar fasciectomy. He has angina, with several episodes of chest pain each week and says that he is 'allergic to local anaesthetics'. Fifteen years ago he had a local anaesthetic block at the dentist, following which he developed palpitations and became very anxious for 10–15 minutes.

Which is the most likely explanation for his previous experience at the dentist?

a **adverse reaction to adrenaline absorbed from the local anaesthetic solution**

b anaphylactic reaction to a preservative in the local anaesthetic solution

c episode of angina brought on by the stress of the situation

d systemic toxicity due to accidental intravascular injection of local anaesthetic

e systemic toxicity due to overdose of local anaesthetic

Most patients with 'LA allergy', particularly after dental surgery, are describing the effects of systemic absorption of adrenaline. It is highly unlikely that enough LA would be injected for a dental block to cause an overdose. Allergy to amide LAs (or their preservatives) is very rare and the symptoms here are not suggestive of an allergic reaction. Although intravascular injection of LA is a possibility his symptoms do not indicate systemic toxicity.

Question 14

An otherwise fit 80-year-old man had uneventful resection of a bladder tumour under general anaesthesia. A three-way irrigating urinary catheter is inserted at the end of the procedure. In recovery, he looks pale and has severe abdominal discomfort. His pulse rate is 48 beats min^{-1} and blood pressure is 75/30. The drained irrigating fluid appears clear.

What is the most appropriate action that would resolve the clinical situation in this patient?

a atropine 0.3 mg IV bolus

b ephedrine 6 mg IV bolus

c **flush the 3–way catheter**

d morphine 5 mg IV bolus

e rapid infusion of 500 ml 0.9% saline

The combination of bradycardia, hypotension, abdominal pain and clear bladder drainage fluid suggests that the patient has bladder clot retention resulting in a vaso-vagal episode. Flushing the catheter is the only action which will resolve this situation.

Question 15

A patient develops anaphylactic shock shortly after induction of general anaesthesia, is treated with intravenous adrenaline and makes an uneventful recovery.

Which is the best explanation of the therapeutic action of adrenaline in the treatment of anaphylaxis?

a causes increased myocardial contractility and bronchodilation

b causes increased myocardial contractility and tachycardia

c **causes peripheral vasoconstriction and decreases mast cell degranulation**

d causes peripheral vasoconstriction and increased myocardial contractility

e causes tachycardia and decreases mast cell degranulation

Decreased mast cell degranulation and peripheral vasoconstriction are the two most important therapeutic actions of adrenaline in the treatment of anaphylaxis.

Question 16

A previously fit 60-year-old woman is oliguric (< 0.5 ml kg^{-1} hr^{-1}) 48 hours after a laparotomy for colonic carcinoma. Laboratory testing of her urine reveals the following:

Specific gravity = 1.020
Sodium 2 mmol L^{-1}
Osmolarity 600 mosmol L^{-1}

What is the most likely diagnosis?

a acute tubular necrosis

b analgesic nephropathy

c **hypovolaemia**

d renal calculi

e bilateral ureteric injury

C is the correct answer. These urinary indices with a high specific gravity, low sodium and high osmolarity are indicative of pre-renal impairment. Hypovolaemia is the only pre-renal cause of the options provided.

Question 17

A 59-year-old man with a caecal carcinoma requiring a right hemicolectomy has been referred for pre-operative assessment. Following an episode of crescendo angina three months previously he had a coronary angioplasty and multiple coronary stent insertion. He is currently well with no further angina and he is taking aspirin and clopidogrel.

What would be the most appropriate management plan for this patient?

a continue both anti-platelet drugs and give a pre-operative platelet transfusion

b postpone surgery until he has completed his anti-platelet therapy

c **schedule urgent surgery and continue both anti-platelet drugs peri-operatively**

d stop aspirin for seven days pre-operatively but continue clopidogrel

e stop clopidogrel for seven days pre-operatively but continue aspirin

Delaying surgery, possibly for many months, is not realistic when treating malignant disease. He is at higher risk of a peri-operative MI if anti-platelet therapy is stopped (due to stent occlusion) than post-operative bleeding. This can be treated with a platelet transfusion if it occurs rather than giving platelets pre-operatively.

Question 18

A 64-year-old man with a BMI of 41 kg m^{-2} had a laparotomy for resection of hepatic metastases one hour ago. In the recovery room his SpO_2 is 85% breathing room air, but 98% when supplemental oxygen is delivered by nasal prongs at 2 L min^{-1}.

Which is the most likely explanation for his current respiratory status?

a alveolar atelectasis

b **alveolar hypoventilation**

c diffusion hypoxia due to nitrous oxide use

d residual neuromuscular blockade

e residual inhalational anaesthesia

Post-operative hypoxaemia is most commonly caused by alveolar hypoventilation, causing a rise in alveolar carbon dioxide. This results in a decrease in the alveolar partial pressure of oxygen, causing peripheral oxygen desaturation. Significant alveolar atelectasis causes true shunt which is not easily improved by inhaled supplemental oxygen administration. C, D and E are unlikely to be significant factors one hour after surgery.

Question 19

Lumbar chemical sympathectomy has a variety of potential therapeutic indications.

Which condition has the best chance of sustained improvement with this technique?

a complex regional pain syndrome type I

b hyperhydrosis

c intermittent claudication

d **ischaemic rest pain in the foot**

e venous ulceration around the ankle

Lumbar sympathectomy can make intermittent claudication worse due to shunting of blood from muscle to skin. Venous ulceration responds poorly (but arterial ulceration well). Sympathectomy results for CRPS are inconsistent and often temporary. Hyperhydrosis does respond but the duration of relief is often transient. Ischaemic rest pain will usually reduce following a chemical sympathectomy (but not the pain from dead tissue!).

Question 20

An 18-year-old male patient is admitted to a district hospital with an isolated severe head injury and is promptly intubated, ventilated and sedated. Soon afterwards his SpO_2 is 99% (FiO_2 0.5), $ETCO_2$ 4.5 kPa, BP 200/120, pulse 44 beats min^{-1} and he has a fixed dilated left pupil.

What is the most appropriate next action to take?

a actively cool the patient to 35°C

b arrange an urgent head CT scan

c arrange transfer to the nearest neurosurgical unit

d insert an arterial line

e **prescribe an intravenous bolus of mannitol 0.5 g kg^{-1}**

The patient is showing signs of severely raised ICP with a marked Cushing's response. Although all of the options are useful in the management of this patient, measures to reduce ICP are urgently required if coning is to be prevented.

Question 21

You are called to the Emergency Department to see a previously well 20-year-old woman who has been admitted following a grand mal fit outside a nightclub. After administration of lorazepam she stops fitting and is now not responsive to commands. Her SpO_2 is 94% on air and blood glucose is 4.5 mmol L^{-1}. No other history is available.

What is the next most useful investigation you would perform on this patient?

a arterial blood gases

b blood alcohol level

c drug toxicology screen

d full blood count

e **serum electrolytes**

A grand mal fit in a previously well patient is unlikely to be due to deranged blood gases or acute alcohol intoxication. Although a toxicology screen would be useful it will take some time to perform. An obvious cause of convulsions has been excluded by a normal blood glucose result. Hyponatraemia secondary to ecstasy ingestion should be considered in this clinical scenario and can be quickly excluded by measuring the serum electrolytes.

Question 22

A 78-year-old woman has had severe, lancinating episodes of pain below the right eye for four months which are sometimes triggered by face washing. Carbamazepine in full doses has produced little improvement in her pain. She has a past history of hypertension and transient ischaemic episodes.

What therapeutic intervention should be considered next?

a **gabapentin**

b microvascular decompression surgery

c slow-release oral morphine

d rhizolysis of the trigeminal ganglion

e amitryptyline

After failure of the first-line treatment for trigeminal neuralgia, gabapentin or microvascular decompression would be the options; in view of the patient's co-morbidities a non-operative approach would be more appropriate for this patient.

Question 23

A previously fit 70-year-old man undergoes radical neck dissection for malignant disease. The patient is stable until the surgeon dissects the tumour away from the carotid sheath. Suddenly, the systolic BP falls from 110 mm Hg to 60 mm Hg, heart rate increases to 110 beats min^{-1}, SpO_2 falls to 87% and end tidal CO_2 concentration falls to 1.9 kPa.

What is the most likely cause for the change in vital signs?

a anaphylactic shock

b carotid sinus manipulation

c myocardial ischaemia

d tension pneumothorax

e **venous air embolism**

Venous air embolism during dissection around the carotid sheath, which contains the internal jugular vein, is the mostly likely cause of the patient's deterioration in this scenario. The patient is likely to be in the head-up position which will increase the risk of air embolism.

Question 24

A previously fit 5-year-old child is distressed and in severe pain in the recovery room following emergency appendicectomy. He is awake and cardiovascularly stable. Intra-operatively, he received fentanyl 3 μg kg^{-1} IV, paracetamol 15 mg kg^{-1} IV and diclofenac 1 mg kg^{-1} PR.

What would be the most appropriate management option now?

a administer Entonox until the child's mother arrives

b codeine phosphate 1 mg kg^{-1} intramuscularly

c codeine phosphate 1 mg kg^{-1} orally

d commence a Nurse-Controlled Analgesia (NCA) pump using morphine

e **morphine 0.1 mg kg^{-1} IV bolus**

The child requires intravenous analgesia – commencing an NCA without a loading dose will be ineffective. The intramuscular route is inappropriate for a paediatric patient; oral medication may not be absorbed due to post-operative ileus.

Question 25

A 26-year-old primigravida (BMI = 47) with a twin pregnancy is in established labour at 38 weeks gestation. She requests an epidural for pain relief but on inserting the epidural needle at L 3, 4 an accidental dural puncture occurs.

What is the most appropriate action to take?

a abandon the epidural and use inhalational analgesia

b abandon the epidural and use opioid-based analgesia

c **insert the epidural catheter intrathecally and use it for spinal analgesia**

d perform an epidural blood patch to prevent post-dural puncture headache

e resite the epidural at an adjacent spinal interspace

A regional block is needed for labour analgesia and the increased possibility of instrumental/operative delivery in the presence of a multiple pregnancy. A further attempt at inserting an epidural is likely to be difficult in view of the patient's high BMI. An epidural blood patch may be required but not during labour.

Question 26

A 70-year-old woman had a gastrectomy 48 hours ago and she has a thoracic epidural for post-operative analgesia which is functioning well. Warfarin, for atrial fibrillation, was stopped seven days ago and she was converted to low molecular weight heparin. Clotting studies and platelet count are in the normal range. Today she is noted to have a white, cold left leg.

What is the most appropriate initial management?

a **doppler studies of the arterial supply of the left leg**

b increase the dose of low molecular weight heparin

c organise an urgent MRI scan of the spine

d top up the epidural with her lying on the left side

e ultrasound of the deep veins of the lower limbs

The patient's history of AF and the clinical findings are highly suggestive of an arterial embolus. The clotting studies are normal which indicates the heparin dosage is sub-therapeutic which has predisposed to the risk of arterial embolism. The priority is to confirm the diagnosis with doppler studies.

Question 27

A 64-year-old man presents to the Emergency Department with an exacerbation of COPD.

His arterial blood gases breathing air show the following:

pH 7.30
pO_2 5.5 kPa
pCO_2 7.5 kPa
HCO_3 35 mmol L^{-1}
Hb 18.5 g dl^{-1}

Which is the most appropriate device to initiate oxygen therapy?

a Hudson mask

b MC mask

c nasal prongs

d non-rebreathing reservoir mask

e **Venturi mask**

The patient's blood gases, with raised bicarbonate and high haemoglobin, indicate that he has long-term severe hypoxaemia and normally retains CO_2. He needs to use a fixed-performance device to ensure that he receives a controlled amount of oxygen as too much oxygen could result in a loss of hypoxic drive and worsening respiratory failure. The Venturi mask is the only fixed-performance device listed.

Question 28

A 35-year-old male suffered a severe isolated traumatic brain injury ten days ago. There is no neurological recovery or respiratory effort 48 hours after cessation of propofol sedation and neuromuscular blockade with atracurium. The serum sodium concentration is 152 mmol L^{-1}, core temperature is 37.5°C; serum glucose concentration is normal. The patient's family know that brain stem death is suspected.

What is the most appropriate action to take now?

a consult the organ donor register

b cool the patient to 36.5°C

c perform an EEG

d reduce serum sodium below 150 mmol L^{-1}

e **undertake brain stem death tests**

The patient has a mild degree of hypernatraemia which is an effect rather than the cause of brain stem death and would not be responsible for the extreme neuro-disability seen in this patient. Mild hyperthermia is not a contraindication to brain stem testing. EEG testing is not part of the brain stem death assessment protocol in the UK.

Question 29

A 70-year-old patient with a long history of severe depression and hypertension is admitted as an emergency with severe peritonitis. He is taking bendroflumethiazide, enalapril and phenelzine. During laparotomy, his blood pressure falls to 65/30 mmHg and heart rate rises to 100 beats min^{-1}. There is no cardiovascular improvement in response to a fluid bolus which raises the CVP to +10 mmHg.

Which is the most appropriate initial pharmacological intervention?

a ephedrine

b metaraminol

c noradrenaline

d **phenylephrine**

e vasopressin

The patient is taking phenelzine which is an MAOI anti-depressant. Drugs with indirect sympathomimetic action are contraindicated in the presence of MAOIs – this excludes ephedrine and metaraminol. Vasopressin and noradrenaline although both directly acting vasoactive drugs would not be considered as first line as they would need to be given as an infusion which would take some time to prepare. A bolus of phenylephrine would be the most appropriate initial response for this severely hypotensive patient.

Question 30

A 19-year-old man is listed for a cervical lymph node biopsy after a six-week history of generalised lymphadenopathy and intermittent pyrexia. He is breathless on mild exertion and needs to sleep with four pillows.

Which is the most important pre-operative investigation that will influence your anaesthetic management?

a CT scan of the neck

b **CXR**

c full blood count

d flow volume loops

e spirometry

The clinical picture indicates a lymphoproliferative malignancy and orthopnoea suggests significant mediastinal involvement, which has major implications for safe general anaesthesia. A CXR would the most useful investigation to initially assess the extent of mediastinal disease.

SOE examination

Clinical Anaesthesia – Long Cases

Case 1

GUIDANCE FOR EXAMINERS

1 Biochemistry results are consistent with mild dehydration.

2 Haematology results show a haemoglobin level of 110 g/L and low platelets.

3 Coagulation screen shows low levels of fibrinogen, prolonged prothrombin time and KCCT.

4 CXR shows pathological changes at the left base, ? due to aspiration.

Topics for discussion
(please spend approximately equal time on each section)

a Pre-operative problems

- Hypovolaemia – assessment (ATLS) – monitoring (CVP, pulse volume variability) – management (what fluids – colloid, blood, FFP and platelets to correct volume and clotting abnormalities) – balance between resuscitation and urgency of surgery
- Renal function – element of renal failure (creat 150 μmol L^{-1} body wt 65 kg) – causes of raised urea – dehydration, renal failure, blood absorption from GIT. Needs catheter, fluid boluses.
- Haematology – needs blood transfusion and correction of clotting and platelet count (NB her platelets may not function because of NSAIDS)
- Respiratory system – consolidation left base ?pneumonia ?aspiration – needs arterial line and blood gases.

b Anaesthesia

- Consent/pre-operative discussion – high chance of requiring post-operative ventilation and ITU care. Opportunity for her to mention resuscitation and end of life care.
- Anaesthetic Plan – RSI (what drugs – smaller induction dose) in theatre fully monitored (pre-induction arterial line)
- Critical incident – loss of cardiac output on induction – Intubate, 100% oxygen, cardiac massage while rapid fluid bolus given, review rhythm (sinus), vasoconstricors (phenylephrine, metaraminol – doses). Causes – hypovolaemia most likely, anaphylaxis possible, cardiac failure (normal rhythm), pulmonary embolus. Responded to fluid and vasoconstrictors.

c Peri-operative managment

- Maintenance of anaesthesia – air/O_2, inhalational agent, atracurium (decreased renal function, but ventilated post-op), opiates. Epidural C/I because – clotting abnormality, urgent surgery, haemodynamically unstable.
- ITU management – chest infection (respiratory care bundle), antibiotics (nosocomial infection more likely e.g. tazocin). Targets for extubation – mentally alert, FiO_2 below 0.5, PEEP +5 cm H_2O, $SpO_2 > 94\%$, respiratory rate < 30 breaths min^{-1}, lactate < 1.5 mmol L^{-1}, normal temperature, decreasing CRP and WBC, low NG aspirate, good analgesia. DVT prophylaxis (?category).
- Feeding options – NG *vs* TPN (pros/cons). Calories/day. Fluid balance. Monitoring response.

Case 2

GUIDANCE FOR EXAMINERS

1 Biochemistry results are normal.

2 Haematology results show haemoglobin 128 g L^{-1} and WBC 13,500 (9,000 polymorphs).

3 CXR shows consolidation of the left lower lobe behind the heart shadow. Peribronchial thickening of the right lower lobe and a large PA are indicative of chronic disease.

a Pre-operative problems

- Review of investigations – normal biochemistry, raised WBC (mainly PMNs). CXR - right looks hyperexpanded because of loss of volume on left. Probable consolidation behind cardiac shadow. Conclusions – likely chest infection
- Respiratory system – management of asthma – ?assessment of severity – accessory muscles, breathless speech, expiratory grunting. SpO_2 helpful. Needs nebuliser and antibiotics (which?) once IV established (Ametop/ EMLA). History of asthma triggers useful.
- Scrotal swelling – differential diagnosis (torsion, viral orchitis, hydrocoele, hernia, trauma, epididymal cyst) – how urgent is surgery? (discuss in view of starvation, full stomach).

b Anaesthesia

- Consent/pre-operative discussion – caudal for post-operative analgesia. What risks would be mentioned – failure, intra-dural/venous injection, infection, weak legs post op. Plan what drug and volume would be used (1 ml kg^{-1} of 0.25% bupivacaine through a cannula).
- Anaesthetic Plan – RSI *vs* normal induction, intubation *vs* LMA (pale, in pain, probable decreased gastric emptying despite vomiting). RSI (drugs, dosages) and ETT used (type, size and length. ? uncuffed protective against aspiration. Take sputum specimen for microbiology.
- Critical incident – sudden rise in inflation pressures when put on ventilator in theatre ? cause e.g. start with patient? Bilateral air entry (exclude pneumothorax and endobronchial intubation), check length of ETT and not kinked, check filter and connections to circuit, check circuit not kinked or trapped, check circuit connected to ventilator correctly, check ventilator settings, check muscle relaxant/depth of anaesthesia.

c Peri-operative management

- Pain relief – limitations of caudal for this (innervation of testis from T12). Morphine 0.1 mg kg^{-1}, paracetamol (15 mg kg^{-1} IV or 30 mg kg^{-1} PR).

?NSAIDS – exacerbation of asthma very rare in children, history useful. Probably use.

- Reversal – dose of glycopyrrolate and neostigmine
- Anti-emetics – which, dose, side effects most encountered.
- Extubation *vs* ITU care – how would you decide? SpO_2 easy to maintain on 35–40% O_2, auscultation, low inflation pressures (below 30 cm H_2O), few secretions up ETT. Assume extubated.
- Post-operative pain relief – ?which regular analgesia. Describe PCA for this age group.

Case 3

GUIDANCE FOR EXAMINERS

1 Haematology results show lowered Hb and raised WBC.

2 Biochemistry results show high normal potassium and raised glucose levels.

3 Arterial blood gas analysis shows a metabolic acidosis.

4 Chest X-ray shows bilateral fractured ribs, surgical emphysema and a chest drain *in situ* on the right.

a Assessment

- Discuss results then proceed to ATLS assessment.
- Airway: Speaking. C spine cleared by CT.
- Breathing: Tachypnoeic – causes – pain, pneumothorax, acidosis, hypovolaemia, flail segment.
- Circulation: estimated blood loss (at least 1.5–2 L).
- Disability – AVPU – is Alert (what are others – Verbal stimulus response, Painful stimulus response or Unresponsive)
- Exposure – other injuries, hypothermia
- What other information needed – AMPLE (allergies, medication, past medical history, last intake, events leading up to injury)

b Resuscitation and Anaesthesia

- Analgesia – may help abdominal assessment. Significance of positive DPL.
- Intubate in A&E *vs* theatres. ? remove collar (safe if no neck pain – CT normal). RSI – discuss drug choices and why. NG tube useful.
- Fluid resuscitation (which fluids and why), blood crossmatch. Monitoring adequacy of resuscitation – ? CVP, urine output, ABGs. Pelvic binder slows bleeding. Transfusion triggers.
- Fluid and body warming important. Risks of inadvertent intra-operative hypothermia (MI in high-risk patients, increased blood loss, increased surgical wound infection, decreased oxygen delivery, altered drug kinetics)

c Peri-operative management

- Respiratory – management of flail chest injury – suggested SV better than IPPV. Problem is underlying lung contusion and infection. CPAP helpful. Pain management options – PCA +NSAIDS, intercostal nerve blocks, interpleural catheter or paravertebral block, epidural, intrathecal opioids. Regional techniques marginally better but not statistically proven.
- Patient not absorbing NG feed after five days post-operatively – investigate and manage – check potassium, CT abdomen, prokinetics-

erythromycin and metoclopramide, consider NJ tube, parenteral nutrition.

- DVT prophylaxis – high-risk use higher dose. Consider warfarin long term.

Clinical Anaesthesia – Short Cases

Paper 1

Question 1: Anaesthetic implications of pacemakers

A 75-year-old man presents for gastrectomy for carcinoma. On pre-operative assessment you find he had a pacemaker fitted three years ago.

How would you proceed?

Supporting information

Nil

How would you proceed?

Pre-operatively ascertain:

1. Pacemaker related:
   - Reason for insertion
   - Pacemaker type
   - Whether has been checked recently
   - Patients underlying rate and rhythm
   - Any clinical features suggesting pacemaker malfunction
   - Information from card, local cardiology dept etc.
2. Evaluate/optimise any other co-existent conditions

Supplementary questions:

1. He has a pacemaker card that says the pacemaker is DDD. What does this mean?

Describes the 'set up' of the pacemaker based on standard international system

- I = Chamber paced (Ventricle, Atrium, Dual)
- II = Chamber sensed (Ventricle, Atrium, Dual)
- III = Mode of response (Triggered, Inhibited, Dual, none)
- IV = Programmable functions (e.g. R – Rate responsive)
- V = Special anti tachycardia functions

2. What are the anaesthetic implications of routine pacemakers?

Physiological effects:

- Variable; e.g. If patient is pacemaker dependant and pacemaker fitted for CHB may have relatively fixed cardiac output

Pacemaker interactions:

- Interaction with diathermy. Use of bipolar if feasible (diathermy may be interpreted as ventricular activity and pacing inhibited)
- (May have to turn off filtering on some ECG monitors to display pacing spikes)
- Have equipment/drugs available in case of pacemaker failure

answer continues/...

3. How does the situation change if the patient has an implantable cardiac defibrillator (ICD) in place because of hypertrophic obstructive cardiomyopathy (HOCM)?

ICD = Implantable device able to detect VF/ VT and deliver electric shocks to terminate. This function must be switched off prior to operation by Cardiology Dept as diathermy may be sensed as shockable rhythm.

Anaesthetic implications of HOCM =

- Keep in sinus rhythm
- Avoid falls in systemic vascular resistance
- Maintain adequate filling to limit left ventricular outflow tract obstruction.

(Filler – How would you manage a failure of a standard pacemaker during the operation?)

Question 2: Septic shock in a patient admitted with cholecystitis.

The outreach nurse calls you for advice regarding a 46-year-old lady admitted to hospital two days previously with acute cholecystitis who is now hypotensive and tachycardic.

What advice would you give?

Supporting information

Arterial blood gases

What advice would you give?

- High likelihood that patient is septic.
- High mortality from severe sepsis (<30%) and incidence increasing. Timely and appropriate intervention can influence outcome (Surviving Sepsis Campaign. Crit Care Med 2004). Patient will need fluid challenge and if remains hypotensive vasoconstrictors and a higher level of care (HDU/ICU) may be required.
- See patient yourself.

What is sepsis?

- Sepsis = presence or suspicion of infection plus two or more of the following (if no infective source it is SIRS):
  - HR > 90
  - RR > 20
  - Temp < 36°C or > 38.3°C
  - WCC < 4 x 10^9 L^{-1} or >12 x 10^9 L^{-1}
- Severe sepsis = sepsis plus evidence of organ dysfunction
- Septic shock = sepsis plus cardiovascular failure defined as systolic BP < 90 mmHg (or a fall of > 40 mmHg) persisting for >30 mins and is unresponsive to fluid boluses (International Sepsis Definitions Conference. *Crit Care Med* 2003).

What is the underlying pathophysiology (briefly)?

- Endotoxin (in the case of gram negative sepsis) triggers an inflammatory cascade of cytokines and adhesion molecules. Complement and clotting pathways are activated. Nitric oxide is released in large quantities.
- This pathway results in vasodilatation, leaky capillaries and a consumptive coagulopathy. The splanchnic circulation is compromised due to diversion of blood to the peripheries and also the presence of microthrombi.
- If left untreated, organ dysfunction occurs and ultimately failure and death.

What would you do when you arrive on the ward?

- Immediate – ABC and monitor response to fluid challenge
- History
  - Has the source of infection been removed (e.g. surgical drain?)
  - Have blood cultures been sent?
  - Have antibiotics been administered?
  - Any relevant comorbidities?
- Examination and chart review
  - RR and SpO_2 (34/min, 92% on 10 L O_2)
  - Current BP/HR (systolic 70 mmHg, HR 192/min)
  - Conscious level (agitated and pulling of facemask)
  - How long has patient been hypotensive (six hours) and what is the MEWS score (12)?

answer continues/...

Investigations?

- Recent FBC and U&E and clotting. Likely to show raised WCC, increasing urea and creatinine, low platelets and raised INR.
- ABG = Primary Metabolic acidosis with respiratory compensation.

Despite receiving several litres of crystalloid the patient remains hypotensive. What would you do?

By definition = septic shock. The patient will require invasive monitoring and vasoconstrictor support (norepinepherine, phenylepherine, vasopressin) to maintain an adequate BP and improve organ perfusion. Although this could be managed in an HDU the severe acidosis with respiratory compromise, the altered GCS and the failure to respond to initial management indicate she is likely to require intubation and therefore transfer to an ICU is required.

- The sepsis care bundle should be implemented which includes
  - Protective ventilation strategies
  - Tight glycaemic control
  - Corticosteroid administration
  - Consideration of activated recombinant human protein C (Xigris)

(Fillers: How may the cardiovascular system be monitored safely and effectively to manage this septic patient in the Intensive Care Unit?)

Key Reference:

Dellinge RP et al. Surviving Sepsis Campaign: International guidelines for management of severe sepsis and septic shock. *Crit Care Med* 2008;**36(1)**:296–327

Question 3: An Obstetric Emergency

You are resident on the Labour Suite. A 23-year-old lady who is 32 weeks pregnant is coming in by emergency ambulance. She was out shopping, went to the toilet and has part of the umbilical cord per vagina.

What would you do?

Supporting information

Nil

What would you do?

Probable diagnosis = cord prolapse

= An obstetric emergency requiring emergency lower segment caesarean section (LSCS)

Management is therefore to prepare for such an event.

Areas to be covered in the initial and supplementary questions:

What would you do prior to her arrival on delivery suite?

- Ensure all interested parties are aware
- Set up theatre/summon senior assistance/liaise with obstetric and neonatal team
- Draw notes if possible

She has now arrived and diagnosis of cord prolapse is confirmed

a) What are your anaesthetic choices?

- Baby needs to be delivered rapidly if ischaemic brain injury is to be avoided
- General anaesthesia probably best option
- Spinal not absolutely contra indicated but with foetal compromise almost certainly present must be rapid

b) What would you do pre-operatively?

- Ensure mother kept head down with manual displacement of presenting part
- Rapid anaesthetic-related history and examination (incl airway)
- Oxygen to mother
- Gain large bore intravenous access (and take bloods – group + save).
- Ranitidine/sodium citrate
- (Rapid foetal assessment by obstetricians)

answer continues/...

Describe the anaesthetic you would undertake for this patient

- Standard check of anaesthetic equipment already done
- Ensure competent anaesthetic assistance
- Induction in theatre on table with obstetric team scrubbed, patient prepped, paediatrician available
- Pre-oxygenation/mandatory monitoring
- Rapid sequence induction with left lateral tilt
- Thiopentone (start 4–6 mg kg^{-1} IV – sleep dose may require more than 6 mg kg^{-1}) and suxamethonium 1–2 mg kg^{-1}. Intubate with appropriate cuffed ET tube. Note: Propofol not licenced for obstetric use.
- Maintenance = Oxygen (in Air or Nitrous oxide), sevo- or iso-flurane (0.5–2 MAC) – adjust to maintain adequate depth of anaesthesia whilst understanding effects on uterine tone
- Following deliver – administer 5 i.u. syntocinon or appropriate infusion (be prepared to discuss the cardiovascular effects oxytocics)
- Prophylactic antibiotics and morphine (0.1 – 0.2 mg kg^{-1} IV) may be given at this stage
- Extubate 'awake' in left lateral position with slight head down tilt

Discuss her post-operative care

- Ideally should be managed initially in a dedicated recovery area
- Continued monitoring, fluids and oxygen by appropriately trained staff
- Analgesia – regular paracetamol and NSAIDs, PCA morphine, bilateral ilioinguinal blocks.

(Filler – The baby is born in poor condition and the paediatricians have not arrived. Describe the assessment and resuscitation of a newborn child.)

Paper 2

Question 1: Anaesthesia for surgery in a patient who is a Jehovah's Witness

You see a patient in the pre-assessment clinic who is a Jehovah's Witness. She is due to have an operative procedure with possible significant blood loss.

What specific problems does this situation pose?

Supporting information

Nil

What specific problems does this situation pose?

- In general, adherents to the faith may not receive allogenic blood transfusions.
- Legally, every competent adult is entitled to refuse to consent to treatment for good reason, bad reason or no reason.
- The patient's wishes must be respected.

Possible supplementary questions:

How would you approach these problems in the pre-assessment clinic?

- Each patient must be assessed individually.
- No absolute rules regarding blood products exist. In general transfusion of blood, FFP and platelets is unacceptable, as is pre-operative autologous blood collection (pre-donation). Blood salvage and fractions of plasma (albumin) may be acceptable.
- Fully document all discussions.
- Consultant-led assessment and care.

What principles apply peri-operatively?

- Pre-operatively – consider staged procedure, use of regional techniques (patient awake) to allow patient to express a change of mind. Check pre-operative haemoglobin concentration, and correct any anaemia before operation.
- Intra-operative – consideration of methods to reduce intra-operative blood loss (e.g. tourniquets, induced hypotension, use of drugs reducing fibrinolysis).
- Post-operative – close monitoring blood loss and reinfusion of blood from drains (knee surgery).

If the patient is 14 years old how would the situation change?

- Complex. Child is of an age where may be 'Gillick competent', i.e. has a clear grasp of the proposed treatment and risks and so can give own consent. He/she may therefore consent to receive a transfusion against parents' wishes. Below 12 or when not competent may need to apply for a 'Specific Issue Order from the High Court' (application to the Court of Session in Scotland).

(Filler – How would the situation change if the patient presented unconscious requiring an emergency operation?)

Key Reference:

Management of Anaesthesia for Jehovah's Witnesses (2nd edition). *AAGBI*, Nov 2005.

Question 2: The child with stridor

You are called to the paediatric ward by your paediatric colleagues to help in the management of a 2-year-old child just admitted with stridor of recent onset. They want your advice on whether the child should be intubated.

How would you assess patency of the airway and the need for intubation?

Supporting information

Nil

How would you assess patency of the airway and the need for intubation?

Clinical assessment based on examination (look, listen, feel)

- Follow ABC approach.
- Assessment of degree of airway obstruction guided by three E's:
  - Effort – Respiratory rate, degree of recession, accessory muscle usage
  - Efficacy – Amount of air movement on auscultation
  - Effectiveness – Mental status, presence of cyanosis, SaO^2, heart rate.
- Need for intubation suggested if hypoxic on high flow oxygen and exhausted. Decision is not a single point decision but involves providing treatment and reassessing.

Possible supplementary questions:

What is stridor?

- High pitched noise, usually inspiratory but may be biphasic if obstruction at tracheal level.

What is your differential diagnosis?

- Infective (viral croup, epiglottitis, bacterial tracheitis)
- Allergy
- Angio-neurotic oedema (itching, facial swelling, rash)
- Trauma
- Inhaled foreign body (sudden onset of coughing, ? choking episode)
- Inhaled hot gases

Describe your initial management?

- High flow oxygen and assessment as above
- Condition specific treatment (e.g. steroid for viral group, adrenaline im for allergy etc, removal under anaesthesia if foreign body suspected)
- Nebulised adrenaline (5 ml 1 in 1,000) buys time
- Regular re-assessment

answer continues/...

The child is toxic (temperature 38.4°C) and unimmunised. There is severe upper airway obstruction. The child is hypoxic but still breathing and you judge intubation is necessary. Describe your anaesthetic approach.

- Senior assistance (Anaesthetic and ENT)
- Transfer to theatre with full airway equipment including cricothyroid puncture set
- No X-rays, sedative premeds or attempts at difficult cannulation
- Gaseous induction (Sevoflorane in oxygen with CPAP as required)
- Cannulation/atropine once consciousness lost
- Airway examination/swabs/antibiotics once deep. Range of uncut tubes available
- Signs of deep anaesthesia = eyes central with small pupils, respiration shallow and diaphragmatic. Once you think the child is deep always wait another five minutes to be sure

(Filler – The airway is lost on induction, and you can neither intubate nor ventilate. How would you manage this?)

SOE **Answers**

Question 3: The lady with bunions

A 72-year-old lady presents for correction of bunions as a day case. On systemic enquiry she complains of aching in the right side of her chest and weight loss of one stone (7 kg) over a three month period. You arrange a pre-operative chest X-ray.

Is the CXR normal?

Supporting information

CXR 3

Is the CXR normal?

- Abnormal CXR. Circumscribed lesion in right mid zone with normal hilum. (Emphysematous changes right upper zone)

Possible supplementary questions:

What is the differential diagnosis?

- Malignancy (95% of cases), rarely hamartoma, Caplan's nodules, AV malformation
- (Diagnosis here was squamous cell carcimona of lung made by CT guided biopsy)

She desperately wants her bunions doing, would you proceed? What would you tell her?

- No. Not in patient's best interests to proceed.
- Your concerns with radiologist.
- Gentle explanation of shadow on the lung requiring further investigation (in presence of spouse/offspring).
- Urgent referral.

She is fully investigated and subsequently listed for an operation involving a thoracotomy (5th rib space). What are the choices for post-operative pain relief after thoracotomy, and their advantages and disadvantages?

- Parenteral opioids
  - – adv = few, disad = poor quality analgesia, cough suppression, PONV
- Epidural analgesia (local anaesthetic plus opioid)
  - – adv = improved quality analgesia, maintain good conscious level plus ability to cough. Aim for thoracic placement. Disad = bilat block, increased nurse supervision required, NAP3 – incidence nerve trauma etc.
- Intrathecal opioids (e.g. single shot preservative-free morphine)
  - – adv = simple. Disad = late respiratory depression, variable effect, supplementary analgesia may be required
- Paravertebral blocks
  - – adv = unilateral block, opioids not required, respiratory function well preserved. Disad = few
- Balanced multimodal approach

How would you manage her airway for such an operation?

- Can be undertaken with a standard ET tube however it helps surgical exposure greatly if use a system that allows one lung ventilation (OLV)
- Usually left-sided double lumen tube
- Confirmation of position (clamping/fibreoptic)
- Problems associated with tube positioning (malposition, specific issues of right-sided tubes, etc.)

(Filler – What are the indications for single lung ventilation?)

Clinical Science

Anatomy

Problems identified at pre-operative assessment

- Hormonal hypersecretion (e.g. Cushing's ACTH, acromegaly GH, prolactinoma, hyperthyroidism thyrotropin)
- Hypopituitarism due to compression by large non-hormone secreting tumour
- Raised intracranial pressure
- Hyperprolactinaemia due to loss of tonic inhibition of prolactin secretion

Problems specific to acromegaly

- CVS: hypertension, LVH, cardiomyopathy with diastolic dysfunction, ECG changes
- Airway: large lips, tongue, face, jaw, OSA, thickening of pharyngeal tissues, laryngeal stenosis
- Also DM, carpal tunnel syndrome

Problems specific to Cushing's disease

- Hypertension with ECG changes
- Obesity, OSA
- Muscular atrophy, myopathy,
- Diabetes mellitus, bruising, osteoporosis

Relevant anatomy of the pituitary

- The pituitary gland or hypophysis is size of a pea
- Sits in the sella turcica (Turkish Saddle) of the sphenoid bone at the base of the middle cranial fossa
- Anterior lobe (adenohypohysis) and posterior lobe (neurohypohysis, releases oxytocin and ADH)
- Linked to the hypothalamus by the pituitary stalk and hypothalamic-hypophyseal portal system
- A portal system means a venous system with capillaries at both ends
- Adenohypophysis hormones are generally under control of hypothalamic releasing hormones
- Enlargement may affect the optic chiasma (temporal or bitemporal hemianopia)
- Mass effect or obstruction of third ventricle may produce increase in ICP
- Lateral extension large tumour may compress cavernous sinuses (cranial nerves III, IV, Vi, Vii, VI pass through so signs are ophthalmoplegia, diplopia, maxillary sensory loss, fixed dilated pupil)

What disorders of serum sodium may be encountered after pituitary surgery

High sodium due to diabetes insipidus (lack of ADH)

- Anti-Diuretic Hormone (aka Arginine Vasopressin) is a nona(9) peptide controls water resorption from cortical and medullary collecting tubules. Acts via aquaporin-2. Action via V2 receptors. V1 – vascular smooth muscle constriction (vasopressin effect).
- Clinical features: polyuria, polydipsia, serum osmolarity > 310 mOsmol L-1, low urine osmolarity.

- Post trauma/ surgical may be triphasic; initial polyuria then antidiuretic phase 4-5 days release of stored hormone). Then permanent DI.
- Treatment: DDAVP (desmopressin). Nasal, IV, IM. Close control of IV therapy/ electrolytes.
- Urine/serum osmolality.
- If some function left; chlorpropamide, clofibrate, carbamazepine.

Low sodium due to SIADH

- Lack of free water clearance so hyponatraemia, hypotonic serum, low urine volumes
- Treat with fluid restriction
- Consider hypertonic saline if Na < 120 mmol L^{-1} with neurological problems
- Raise serum Na slowly to avoid central pontine myelinolysis
- Demeclocycline use is described
- Newer V1/ V2 receptor blockers tolvaptan, conivaptan now advertised for treatment SIADH

Physiology

Cardiac effects:

- Sudden ↑ afterload and SVR (40%), ↓ venous return, SV and CO (15–30%)
- Affects on blood pressure may be variable due to opposing effects of SVR and CO
- May need drugs to control BP (vasodilators – SNP, GTN, and/or inotropes)
- If pre-existing IHD, often acute left ventricular failure:
- Large fall in SV, big increase in PAOP, arrhythmias, subendocardial ischaemia
- worse if suprarenal clamp, increase in; MAP, PAOP, wall motion abnormalities, ↓ LVEF
- identify patients at risk pre-op, early use of vasodilators
- GTN preserves transmural blood flow, reduces ↓ in contractility, SNP may cause 'steal'
- If SV, CO, SvO_2 low after GTN, with normal PAOP, consider inotropes (amrinone)

Renal:

- Decreased RBF, GFR, urine output, even with infrarenal clamping
- renal vascular reflexes following clamping, embolised atheromatous material, trauma to kidney?
- Not prevented with use of epidural anaesthesia to T6
- 3–14% acute renal failure, no protection with frusemide, mannitol or dopamine

Spinal cord damage:

- Due to damage to infrarenal radicular arteries or anomalous artery of Adamkowitz
- More common with high clamp, 5–40% paraplegic
- Protection tried with barbiturates, NMDA antagonists, magnesium, calcium antagonists, hypothermia, CSF drains to reduce CSF pressure and maintain cord perfusion

Metabolic changes:

- Ischaemia of muscle, bowels, anaerobic metabolism, lactic acidosis, vasomotor paralysis, vasodilatation

What is meant by reperfusion injury and what is the mechanism?

- **Direct** injury caused during the ischaemic interval, due to hypoxia
- **Indirect** injury that occurs during reperfusion >
- Injury produced by reperfusion is *greater* than that due to ischaemia, affects all organs
- Lactate washed out from limb > vasodilatation and afterload reduction
- During ischaemia, hypoxanthine formed. On reperfusion xanthine oxidase catalyses reaction between hypoxanthine and oxygen to xanthine and an oxygen free radical (superoxide)
- Free radicals cause membrane damage, impair protein synthesis, and activate neutrophils and result in release of cytokines (IL-1, IL-6, IL-8,TNF alpha)
- Neutrophils adhere to microvascular endothelium and migrate into tissues
- Neutrophils contain NADPH oxidase that produces more oxygen free radicals (i.e. cascade)
- Cytokines initiate an inflammatory response affecting renal, CVS, RS, CNS, leading to MODS

Some areas of anaesthetic best-practice in open aortic surgery

- Monitoring: IABP, CVP, TOE, PAFC, temperature, SpO_2, ABGs, blood loss, urine out etc.
- Avoid hypovolaemia: full and dilated circulation at reperfusion (? benefit of thoracic epidural use)
- Cross-clamp time: longer cross-clamp times cause more ischaemic problems (up to 30 mins acceptable)
- Staged reperfusion: release of arteries phased (L and R internal and external iliac in turn)
- Aorto-femoral shunt: to reduce ischaemia may be used
- Cardiopulmonary bypass for thoracic aorta
- Reactive oxygen species scavengers i.e. drugs that ↓ impact of reperfusion injury

Pharmacology

Features of LA toxicity

CNS:

- Visual and hearing disturbances, tingling in tongue, lips, dizziness, tinnitus. dysarthria, disorientation, muscle twitching and rigidity
- Loss of consciousness, fits (increased if hypercarbia), coma, respiratory arrest

CVS: Racemic bupivacaine> Laevo bupivacaine/Ropivacaine

- Arrhythmias, increased PR interval/QRS duration– inhibition of normal conduction (blocks Na+ channel)
- Ventricular dysrhythmias due to re-entry circuit resulting from slowed conduction
- Initial ↑ systolic and diastolic/BP, Negative inotrope (due to ↓ intracytoplasmic calcium), ↓ ejection fraction, increase in pulmonary artery pressures
- Falls in tissue pH with CVS collapse worsen effects with bupivacaine

What are the factors which determine whether LA toxicity develops

Operator factors:

- Mass of drug given (relative to patient size) – total more important than concentration
- Speed of injection

Site of injection:

- depends on vascularity (intercostals>epidural>plexus>peripheral)

Pharmacological factors:

- Potency of drug (bupivacaine x4 potency of lignocaine)
- Protein binding. In plasma mainly alpha-1 glycoprotein, high affinity, low capacity
- Only 'buffers' changes. Tissue protein binding reduces drug availability
- Clearance, by redistribution, elimination and metabolism

What is the mechanism of action of LA toxicity

- Injected into tissues, physiological pH 7.4, increase in unionized form, more lipophilic, crosses cell membrane
- Intracellular pH lower (7.1), increase in ionization, blocks Na+ channel from within (binding to domain IVS6 charged molecule in pore → electrostatic repulsion rather than physical block) (Na+ channel must be open)
- Na channels can be closed , open or inactivated. Both R and S block open channels but block of inactivated Na channels is stereospecific R(+) Bupivacaine doing so faster and with more potency. 'Fast-in-slow-out'
- 9 Sub groups of human Na channels with αα changes in α/β subunits → differing binding affinities
- Unionized portion may also block Na+ channel via membrane, does not rely on Na+ channel being open

Management of systemic bupivicaine toxicity (AAGBI Guidelines updated 2010)

- ABC
- Intralipid (20%) – mechanism unclear , concept of 'lipid sink'. Immediately 1.5 ml/ kg over one minute and infusion at 15 ml kg^{-1} hr^{-1}. After five mins repeat maximum two boluses, can double infusion rate

Describe LA structure and factors affecting activity

- Aromatic or benzene ring – lipophilic; weak bases, pKa ~ 8 (lidocaine 7.9, bupivacaine 8.1)
- Linked by ester or amide bond to tertiary amine with side-chain – hydrophilic.
- Bup/Rop this amine is piperidine ring, containing chiral carbon atom, plus butyl/ propyl sidechain
- Ester or amide bond, esters metabolized by plasma esterases, amides in liver
- Prepared as HCl salts, pH in ampoule low, predominantly ionized/water soluble (active)
- Lipid solubility. Increases penetration of membrane. Higher solubility, greater potency, increased rate of onset, longer duration of action
- pKa. Lower pKa, more unionized at body pH (i.e. rapid onset). At any given pH, more bupivacaine ionized compared with lidocaine. LAs do not work well in infected (acidic) tissues
- Protein binding. Reduces availability (slows onset), but increases binding to membrane proteins prolonging duration

Clinical measurement

Sources of pollution by anaesthetic vapours and gases

- Insufflation techniques, gas induction, spillage, leaks, facemasks, LM, T-piece, monitors gas sampling vents, post-anaesthetic exhalation of vapour, failure to turn off vapour/gas flow after anaesthesia etc.

Concerns

- Reports of increased abortion rates, increased rates of malignancy, decreased fertility, mortality
- Personnel particularly at risk: paediatric anaesthetists, bronchoscopists, recovery staff, etc.

Nitrous oxide

- Occupational exposure limit to nitrous oxide in the UK is 100 ppm over an eight hour time weighted average
- Below 100 ppm there is no evidence of increased risk of malignancy, or decreased fertility in exposed staff, although risk of spontaneous abortion might be slightly increased
- Prolonged exposure to high concs. N2O causes megaloblastic bone-marrow depression and ↓ DNA synthesis

Isoflurane

- Chronic exposure to trace concentrations of isoflurane may cause dose-dependent genetic damage, (comparable with smoking 11–20 cigarettes a day) and a derangement in lymphocyte subpopulations
- Current COSHH recommendations for isoflurane = 50 ppm over eight hour time weighted average

How may anaesthetic gas pollution be reduced or prevented?

- Use TIVA O_2/air
- Consideration of use of N_2O and gaseous anaesthetics (particularly for induction). If need to use > low flows
- Ensure operating theatres are efficiently ventilated (minimum 15 exchanges/hour)
- Keyed fillers for vaporisers
- *Scavenging* when using gaseous anaesthesia is an essential element in the control of exposure

Features of a scavenging system

- *Passive:* patient dependent, no active +ve or –ve pressure > 30 mm connector> reservoir + value to protect against excessive pressure effects, low resistance (< 0.5 cm H_2O) at 30 L min^{-1}). Rarely used in modern theatres
- *Active*: pumped waste removal, collecting system > tubing > reservoir (protected against –ve pressures etc > disposal system (fan or ejector). Active scavenging must not extract patient fresh gas, etc.

Other reasons for efficient ventilation

- Laminar flow
- Air within a designated space moves with uniform velocity in a single direction along parallel flow lines, is usually restricted to an area in the centre of the operating theatre (room within a room principle)
- Laminar air flow can be used to create an ultra-clean environment, and is recommended for prosthetic implant surgery: this system provides over 400 air changes per hour by recirculating air after passing it through high-efficiency filters (0.5 μm)
- All ventilation systems should provide a positive pressure across any openings, so that when doors are opened there is less chance of bacterial egress
- Opening of doors and other movement makes the system less efficient (opening theatre door displaces 2 m^3 of air into theatre)

Other environmental factors to consider in theatre design:

- Temperature control – patient cooling, staff comfort and fatigue, evaporative losses, neonates, etc.
- Humidity controlled to 40–60% (why?)